# Atlas of stomal pathology

*I tell you that which you yourselves do know,*
*Show you sweet Caesar's wounds, poor poor dumb mouths,*
*And bid them speak for me.*

William Shakespeare
(Julius Caesar, Act III, sc. II)

Antonello Franchini, M.D., F.I.C.S.
Professor of Surgery
Director of the Institute of Surgical Semeiotic
Bologna University School of Medicine
Bologna, Italy

Bruno Cola, M.D., F.I.C.S.
Associate Professor of Surgery
Senior Registrar of the Institute of Surgical Semeiotics
Bologna University School of Medicine
Bologna, Italy

Priscilla J. d'E. Stevens, S.R.N.
Principal Stomatherapist
Groote Schuur Hospital
Cape Town, South Africa

*With special contributions by:*

Professor A. Montagnani
Director of the Dermatological Clinic
University of Bologna
Bologna, Italy

*and*

Professor A. Martelli
Director of the Urological Clinic
University of Bologna
Bologna, Italy

Preface by Professor B. N. Brooke, M.D., M. Chir., F.R.C.S., Hon. F.R.A.C.S., London

# Atlas of stomal pathology

by
A. Franchini
B. Cola
P.J.d'E. Stevens

*Preface by Prof. B.N. Brooke*

With 353 full-colour illustrations

A CORTINA MEDICAL PUBLICATION

cortina international · verona
distributed by
Raven Press/New York

CORTINA INTERNATIONAL - VERONA
*a branch of*
EDIZIONI LIBRERIA CORTINA VERONA S.r.l.
Via C. Cattaneo, 8 - 37121 Verona (Italy) - Tel. 045/38821-594818 - Telex 431107 CORTIN I

© Copyright 1983
ISBN 88-85037-37-2

First English Edition 1983
Published simultaneously in Italian language

Translated from the Italian by A. Steele

Printed in Italy by Edizioni Libreria Cortina Verona
Via C. Cattaneo, 8 - 37121 Verona (Italy)

# CONTENTS

# PREFACE

*Stomas have to be seen to be believed – that is why this atlas is such a timely and valuable addition to the growing literature on an advancing subject; for stoma problems all too often beggar description. The few stoma patients, articulate enough to speak about their orifice, have a descriptive language of their own which can sometimes be helpful. But for communication within medicine – from doctor to doctor, nurse to nurse and most important nurse to doctor – this is clearly imprecise and will not suffice. Professor Franchini, Professor Cola and Sister Stevens have therefore chosen photographic illustration as the hieroglyph to implement their work. It was, in fact, a post hoc decision since it has been their practice to illustrate case records; review of these records has caused them to become aware of the considerable need for information to be disseminated in no uncertain way regarding stoma failure. What could be better than an atlas of high quality with illustrations which catch the eye?*

*The need has arisen, not so much because colostomy, ileostomy or urostomy have intrinsic defects; quite the reverse – properly constructed, they are efficient alternatives to their natural counterparts, provided, that is, that they are properly managed. There's the rub; even in this day and age of stoma care, patients all too often leave hospital ill equipped with the means and the know-how. The trouble lies in the fact that stoma care is still a speciality, certainly in nursing terms and to a not much lesser degree in medicine. The speciality arose ironically not with the original stoma, for any Tom, Dick or Harriet could get by more or less with a colostomy; it was born of the complexities of ileostomy management, and since this stoma only came into established practice after Koenig's invention of the adherent bag in 1944, it has only become a part of surgical routine in recent times. New generations of doctors and nurses are entering practice who take these matters in their stride because they have encountered them in their training; there are, nevertheless, more senior cadres to whom stoma care is new and foreign territory. Therefore patients can still leave hospital without the advice they need and, regrettably, even with a poorly constructed stoma.*

*The experience of the authors is based upon a wealth of such cases; being well known in the field, it has been their lot to attract difficult problems. In producing this work they have done a particular service; it will help to spread knowledge and restore stoma care to where it should belong – in general nursing and general medicine, although the construction of urostomies and of continent stomas should, because of their complexity, remain in specialist hands. It is the responsibility of pioneers to create a general awareness; the three authors will achieve that admirable aim with the Atlas of Stomal Pathology.*

BRYAN N. BROOKE
M.D., M. Chir., F.R.C.S., Hon. F.R.A.C.S
Emeritus Professor uf Surgery
University of London, St. George's Hospital

# ACKNOWLEDGEMENTS

*The authors wish to express their sincerest thanks to all those who in different ways have made this work possible: the Department of Surgical Semeiotics of the St. Orsola University Hospital, Bologna; the Department of Surgery, including the Urological and Paediatric Sections, of the Groote Schuur Hospital, Cape Town; Professor A. Lennox-Short, M.A., F.R.S.A.; Mrs. Franca Masi and Mrs. Umberta Fraschi, stomatherapists in the Bologna University Department of Semeiotics; the Department of Clinical Photography of the Groote Schuur Hospital and the Red Cross Children's Hospital.*

*Our thanks also go to Professor B.N. Brooke for his highly flattering Preface, Coloplast A/S for their unstinting contribution and Chirurgica S.p.A. for their unfailing support.*

*A special acknowledgement is due to our understanding patients, who, by allowing themselves to be photographed, have become the true protagonists of this atlas.*

# Atlas of stomal pathology

# 1. Introduction

Before he writes a book, an author needs, first of all, a basic idea. Then he must develop it in accordance with his background and experience.

When he sets about compiling an atlas, his basic idea is not enough. He needs photographs. He can collect them as they come his way or he may have to go out of his way to find them and, sometimes, to photograph or have photographed what is arranged rather than fortuitous.

This was not how this atlas came into being. The idea came to us subsequently. We suddenly realised, out of the blue, that our habit of documenting everything we had observed had yielded a whole wealth of photographic material on the subject.

The series, dealing, as it does, with poorly constructed or diseased stomata, might not, at first sight, have seemed very exciting and might, in fact, have appeared rather repetitive. But a moment's thought was enough to convince us that reactions to the material in question would have been quite different, had they been those of the people directly concerned: the ostomy patients themselves.

The stoma is in fact, an organ which is part and parcel of the body. The ostomy patient comes to regard it as he does his liver or stomach, and there can be no doubt that it deserves far more attention than has been devoted to it.

It is a new organ with its own particular anatomy, that determined by the surgeon, its own physiology closely, but not exclusively, linked to the digestive apparatus and its own varied, all too frequent pathology.

The subject matter, therefore, is in no way insignificant. It seems to be so merely because of a tendency to belittle its importance because of the limited interest shown in it in scholarly medical circles.

The truth is that, in treatises on surgical pathology, stomal affections are ignored or are dismissed in a few lines. But when dealing with surgical techniques, authors describe at great length the methods used to construct stomata while there are many studies on their function.

This gap in our documented knowledge is unjustified and, indeed, inexcusable. Stomata can give rise to a multiplicity of disorders, while various forms of stomal pathology may cause both acute suffering and very severe limitations. Furthermore, such problems are all too often the results of the errors or even the minor inaccuracies of which the surgeon is guilty when making the stoma.

Yet, in itself, the technique is not difficult to master, and, even with the great variety of stomata available,

one cannot go far wrong if one keeps to a number of simple, standard procedures applicable in all cases; choice of a loop which is definitely healthy and adequately mobilised (Fig. 1.1); scrupulous care in performing the viscero-parietal fixation (Fig. 1.2 A, B, C); skin incision separate from the main incision and always of the disk-removal type for terminal stomata (Fig. 1.3 A, B, C); careful mucocutaneous fixation with or without eversion according to the portion of bowel used (Figs. 1.4 and 1.5).

Thus it is by no means easy to understand why so many stomata are poorly constructed, while it is disconcerting to note the inadequate attention paid to the disturbances which such stomata give rise to in addition to the spontaneous stomal pathology, which can make life difficult enough for the ostomy patient.

Recently these problems have come to the fore because of a substantial increase in the number of ostomy patients. Their rehabilitation has become an imperative necessity and the social methods of achieving this are being applied throughout the world.[85]

Ostomy patients are gradually realizing that their limitations do not result so much from their having a stoma, as from the fact that the stoma they have may be poorly constructed or even diseased.

The frequency, variety and seriousness of stomal pathology and the need to cure it, convinced us that

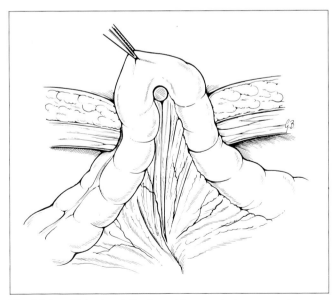

**Fig. 1.1.** Insufficient mobilization of the exteriorised loop: the result is abdominal wall retraction and risk of detachment. The stoma proves difficult to manage.

1

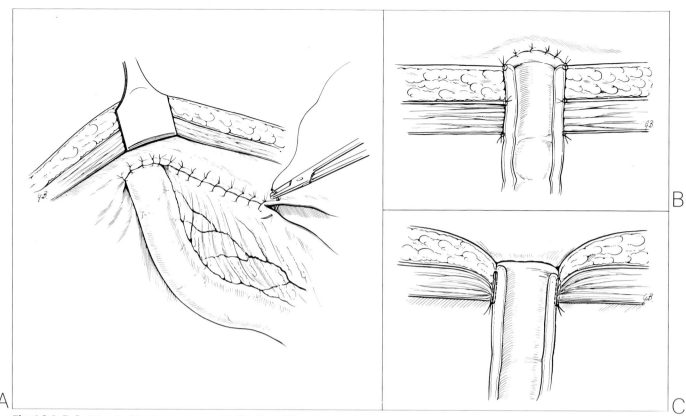

**Fig. 1.2 A, B, C.** A) Lack of fixation or incomplete fixation of the mesentery to the parietal peritoneum results in internal hernia and prolapse. Fixation along the parietal route, which is optional, should respect the various layers (B) and not bunch them up (C), otherwise there will be retraction.

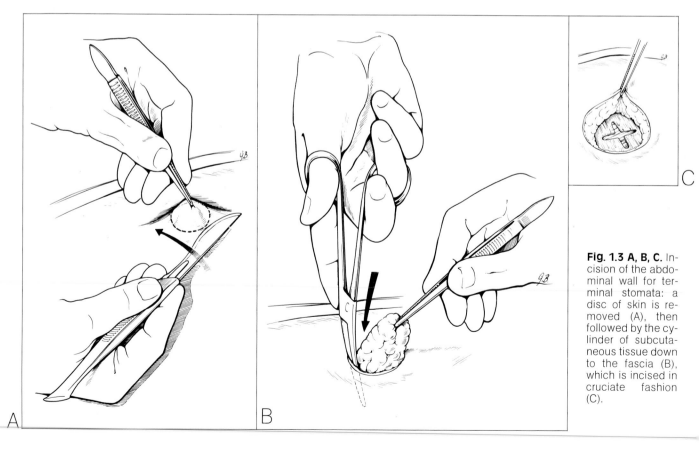

**Fig. 1.3 A, B, C.** Incision of the abdominal wall for terminal stomata: a disc of skin is removed (A), then followed by the cylinder of subcutaneous tissue down to the fascia (B), which is incised in cruciate fashion (C).

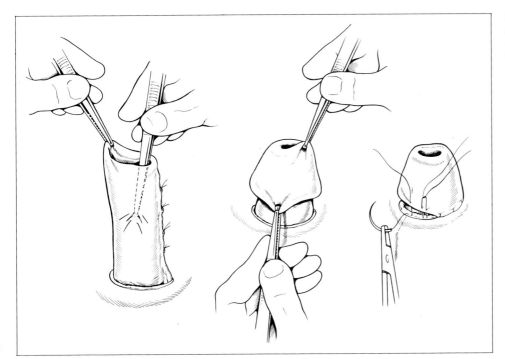

**Fig. 1.4.** Ileostomy with eversion according to the traditional technique. It will be noted that the mucocutaneous suture is confined to the derma.

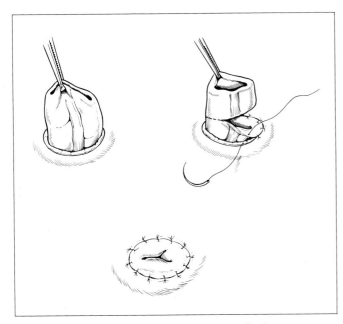

**Fig. 1.5.** Colostomy with flat mucocutaneous fixation.

something had to be done to bring order into this field of study. This is precisely what we set out to achieve with this atlas. There was no lack of the experience necessary for such a task. This is indicated by the abundance of photographic material. It is all original and pertains to diseases either operated on or observed and treated medically by the stomatherapy services of the Bologna University Institute of Surgical Semeiotics and of the Groote Schuur Hospital, Cape Town.

In addition to our experience, the atlas benefits from the most recent literature on the subject and the collaboration of two eminent specialists, Professors Martelli and Montagnani.

We must also mention the invaluable contribution made to this work through documents such as those kindly provided by Professors Standerskjöld-Nordenstam and Waye.

The reader will, of course, judge the value of the work for himself. As far as we, the authors, are concerned, our point will have been made if, on turning over the pages of this atlas, surgeons convince themselves (if they have not already done so) of the need to devote more serious attention to stomal pathology and its prevention whenever they construct a stoma.

# 2. Clinical examination of the ostomy patient

In very few categories of patients does the clinical examination require more time and care than in an ostomy patient.

It is not enough just to check the functioning of his stoma or ascertain the existence of any impaired function; one has to assess the repercussions which the loss of a portion of bowel has on the entire organism, verify the degree to which the ostomy patient has mastered the techniques of stoma management and, lastly, carry out the appropriate checks with regard to his original disease or condition.

If to all this we then add the innumerable psychological difficulties which afflict even the more fortunate of ostomy patients, it will be readily appreciated that the contact which has to be established with the ostomy patient is of a very particular nature and involves a thoroughly frank and detailed exchange of views based, on the one hand, on the stomatherapist's understanding and positive disposition towards the patient and, on the other, on the patient's confidence in the stomatherapist.

The elements which emerge in the course of each visit should be noted on personal record cards with a view to assessing the basic trend of the ostomy patient's situation as well as the variations in that situation over time. It is, however, essential to temper one's cold, strictly technical approach with a humanitarian attitude; the results of rehabilitation depend equally upon these two components.

## Case history

A thorough knowledge of the clinical history is of great assistance when caring for an ostomy patient.

In the course of the first visit it is therefore good policy to ask the patient about past pathological events and about the disease or condition which necessitated the construction of the stoma. One needs to have a precise idea as to what the patient actually knows about the original disease and not be over-hasty in revealing to him certain truths of which he may be unaware before one has had time to obtain a perfectly clear picture of his psychological characteristics.

One then goes over to the actual case history as such, enquiring as to the patient's life style, diet, culture and social aspirations.

On completing the general picture, one now procedes to gather data as to the functioning of the stoma and any variations in its morphology.

The case history is concluded by inviting the ostomy patient to indicate all the particular or general problems troubling him, filling in the gaps in his account by means of specific questions aimed at exploring those aspects which he has deliberately omitted to clarify or has overlooked.

It may, however, be good policy in this context to put off delicate investigations such as those relating to sexual activities to a later meeting when a greater degree of familiarity has been established.

## General physical examination

Once the ostomy patient is lying on the examination couch and the stomatherapist has performed the preparatory manoeuvres of removing the stoma appliance and cleansing the skin, it is unwise to go straight ahead with the examination of the stoma as this may reinforce the patient's impression that he is there for that reason alone.

A better policy is to proceed with a careful general examination with particular reference to the possible effects of the operation on the organism as a whole as well as to any possible recurrence of the original disease.

Special attention should therefore be paid to the state of hydration, the trophism of the tissues and the sanguification conditions in colectomy patients, especially those who have undergone an ileal resection, and one should perform palpation of the abdomen, liver and lymph nodes in patients operated on for carcinoma.

If there is a residual ampulla of the rectum, this should be explored digitally and examined endoscopically; conversely, if the patient has been subjected to amputation of the rectum, one procedes to examine the perineum.

## Examination of the stoma

This is performed on the basis of inspection and palpation.

The inspection enables one to assess the diameter, colour and degree of protrusion of the stoma in addition to the condition of the peristomal skin.

The diameter, which is gauged with special measuring devices (Fig. 2.1), is extremely important, inasmuch as variations in the stomal diameter may be the first sign of numerous pathological events.

As regards the colour, one has to assess any differences in relation to the characteristic colour of healthy bowel mucosa.

It is, of course, impossible to use fixed reference pa-

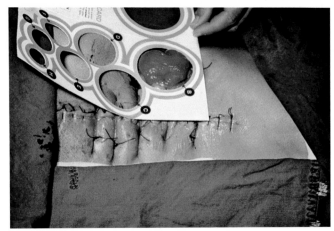

**Fig. 2.1.** Measuring the stomal diameter.

2.6). The differential diagnosis is not difficult and is based on the consistency of the stomal mucosa, which, in ischaemia, resembles the consistency of cardboard, whereas in melanosis it is normal, as well as on the tendency towards visceroparietal detachment which is a constant feature of acute vascular distress.

As far as the degree of protusion is concerned, if this is greater than 3-4 centimetres in an ileostomy or even less in a colostomy, it is an indication of prolapse, while a reduction in the degree of protrusion inclines us towards a diagnosis of retraction. In these cases it is indispensable to know the initial length of the stoma because what matters are the variations in this length.

The other element which is detectable by inspection is the state of the peristomal skin.

Apart from the immediate ascertainment of the pres-

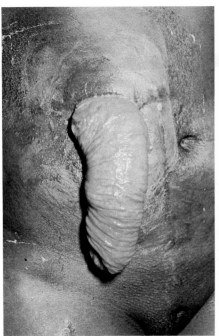

**Fig. 2.2.** Prolapsed transverse colostomy in young African female suffering from severe anaemia.

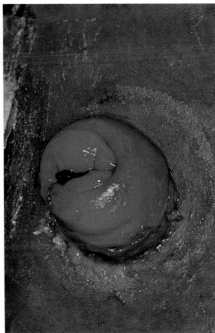

**Fig. 2.3.** Ileostomy, bright red in colour, due to congestion and hyperaemia in young African male suffering from acute enteritis.

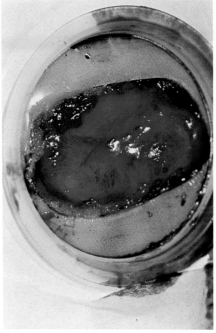

**Fig. 2.4.** Colostomy, dark red in colour, severely congested and bleeding, in a septicaemic patient.

rameters, and, moreover, account must be taken of the emotionally induced hyperaemia often occasioned by the examination itself. Nevertheless, just as a pale stoma is characteristic of severe anaemia (Fig. 2.2), a congested, hyperaemic stoma with a clearly visible vascular network (Fig. 2.3) indicates the presence of enteritis or inflammatory colopathy.

Shades of darker red with accentuation of the congestion accompanied by bleeding (Fig. 2.4) are characteristics of a state of severe, generalized sepsis.

Cyanosis, which indicates an initial state of venous distress, manifests itself in the form of dark, bluish or purple patches (Fig. 2.5).

Lastly, the black colour, when it is not an expression of severe ischaemia, is due to the presence of melanosis of the colon used in constructing the stoma (Fig.

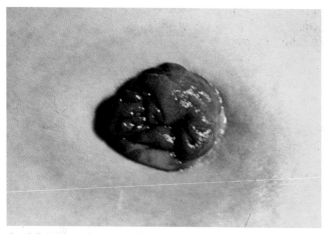

**Fig. 2.5.** Right colostomy with purple patches, typical of cyanosis.

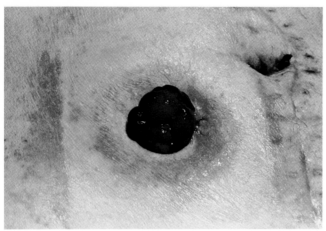

Fig. 2.6. Ileo-caecal loop urinary diversion with intense melanosis.

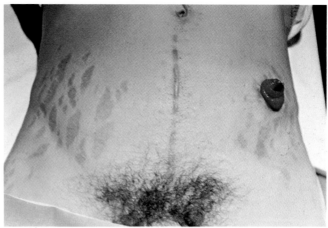

Fig. 2.7. Striae of the abdominal skin in a colostomy patient who had suffered from nephrotic syndrome and had lost more than 30 kg in weight. The use of simple adherent colostomy bags could cause serious dermatitis in the striae sites.

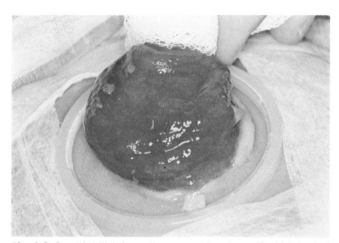

Fig. 2.8. Small whitish formations on an ileostomy. On histological examination, they turn out to be Peyer's plaques.

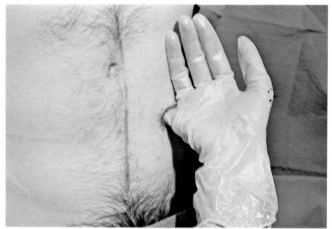

Fig. 2.9. Digital examination of the stoma.

ence of dermatitis, one should also assess the trophism, elasticity, dryness and pigmentation of the skin. In addition, one should also take account of any skin disorders which, though they may be independent of the stoma, may nevertheless interfere with stoma management (Fig. 2.7).

Lastly, it is worth recalling that observation of the stoma may reveal neoformations of the mucosa, the nature of which must be ascertained by means of a biopsy (Fig. 2.8). This is performed with great care by means of a tangential section or wedge resection. Haemostasis must be achieved by cauterization or by suture.

The second phase of the stomal examination, after performing palpation of the region in search of a possible hernia, consists in digital exploration of the stoma, using the lubricated, gloved little finger (Fig. 2.9).

The elasticity of the stomal orifice, the internal diameter of the lumen at both skin fascial level and the angle formed by the bowel and abdominal wall are assessed.

It is thus possible to detect the onset of stenosis or the presence of extrinsic compression on the stomal loop.

On withdrawing the finger, the latter must be observed in order to detect the presence of streaks of blood just as in rectal examination.

The examination should be completed by assessing the quality of the motions, and to this end one observes the contents of the bag worn by the ostomy patient.

Special attention should be devoted to particular sto-

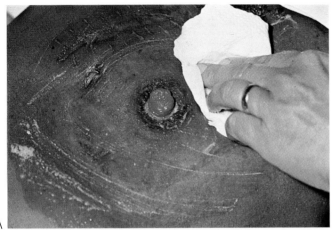

A

mata such as an ileal or a colonic conduit, continent ileostomies and magnetic colostomies.

In the case of urinary conduit, the stoma is slightly dilated so as to ensure that there is no stenosis with subsequent pooling, and urine samples may be taken and sent to the laboratory (Fig. 2.10 A, B, C).

Patients with a continent ileostomy should be asked to perform a catheterization so as to check the functioning of the valve (Fig. 2.11).

Patients with magnetic colostomies should have the position of the magnetic ring checked with the special instrument designed for the purpose (Fig. 2.12).

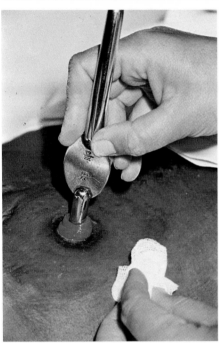

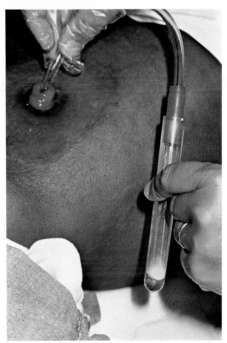

B

**Fig. 2.10 A, B, C.** All management procedures relating to a urinary diversion should be performed in conditions of maximum sterility. A) Disinfection of the peristomal skin with bacterial solutions. B) Delicate dilatation of the stoma with sterile instruments. C) Taking a urine sample in sterile conditions.

C

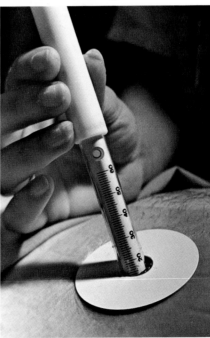

**Fig. 2.12.** Checking the position of the ring in a magnetic colostomy by means of the use of a special instrument for the purpose.

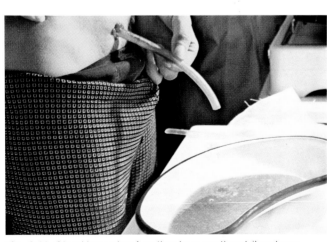

**Fig. 2.11.** Checking valve function in a continent ileostomy.

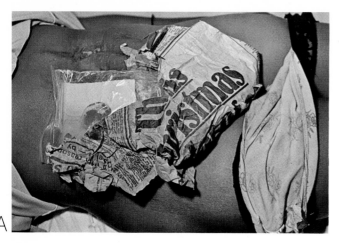

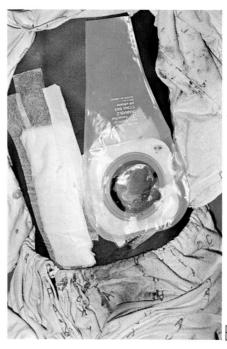

**Fig. 2.13 A, B.** Two examples of unorthodox management in patients unable to master conventional stoma care: A) Newspaper. B) Bag upside down and failure to apply closure clamp.

## Assessment of the extent to which the ostomy patient has mastered the stoma management techniques

Apart from exceptional cases associated with particular social and cultural conditions (Fig. 2.13 A, B), the ostomy patient to-day, providing he has been properly

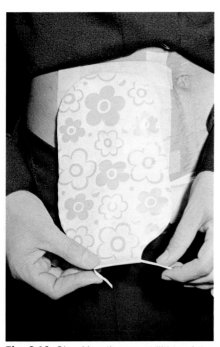

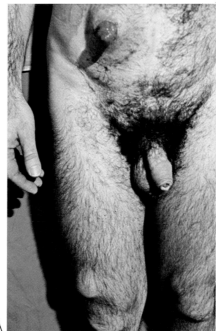

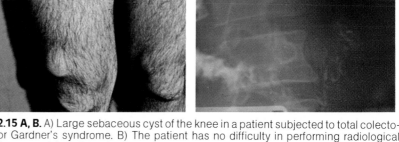

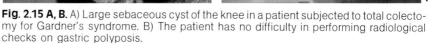

**Fig. 2.14.** Checking the capabilities of the ostomy patient.

**Fig. 2.15 A, B.** A) Large sebaceous cyst of the knee in a patient subjected to total colectomy for Gardner's syndrome. B) The patient has no difficulty in performing radiological checks on gastric polyposis.

instructed before being discharged from hospital, is perfectly capable of managing his stoma by himself.

Nevertheless, it is good policy to check the extent to which he has mastered the stoma management techniques by asking him questions about cleansing and appliance management procedures.

Should doubts arise, it is a good idea to ask him to perform these manoeuvres (Fig. 2.14), correcting him even in minor details.

Colostomy patients who practise irrigation, – especially those who complain of unsatisfactory results – should be asked to demonstrate the wash-out procedures in precise detail. Account should be taken of the various individual modifications which any ostomy

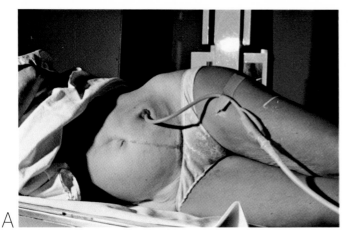

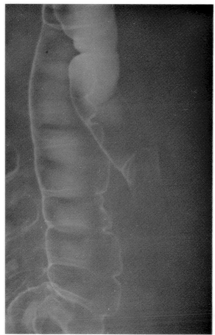

Fig. 2.16 A, B. A) Barium enema may be performed in an ostomy patient using a normal balloon probe. B) The radiological result is well-nigh perfect.

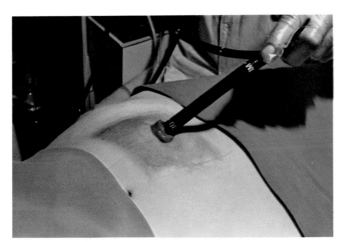

**Fig. 2.17.** Colonoscopy via a colostomy.

## Supervision of the original disease

The presence of a stoma does not prevent us from performing the radiological and instrumental investigations normally undertaken for diseases of the abdominal organs.

The ostomy patient may thus undergo a radiological examination of the alimentary tract (Fig. 2.15 A, B) without having to adopt any special techniques or may be given a barium enema, special probes[28, 29] or standard balloon catheters being used to prevent the discharge of contrast medium and air from the stoma (Fig. 2.16 A, B).

Colostomy patients who practise irrigation do not need to undergo any particular preparation of the bowel, whereas the others may adopt the method preferred by the radiologist without any drawbacks. It proves just as easy to perform endoscopies (Fig. 2.17), and here, too, there are no difficulties as regards bowel preparation.

All other investigations – ultrasonography, scintigraphy and computerized axial tomography, to mention but a few – may be performed without the presence of the stoma giving rise to difficulties.

patient tends to make in relation to the standard techniques according to his physical characteristics and life habits. It is impossible to list these, because in this field colostomy patients exercise a very high degree of ingenuity and imagination, devising solutions capable of astonishing even the shrewdest and most experienced stomatherapist.

# 3. Primary stomal pathology

This chapter covers two groups of stomal diseases. The diseases of the first group, which may be termed congenital, are characterized by a defect of primary formation, be it an actual technical error such as a poor choice of site or a surgical mishap as in the case of ischaemia or suppuration. The second group, which includes granulomas, traumas abd skin lesions, may be defined as acquired diseases of various origins.

All these diseases may be manifested right from the time the stoma is constructed or may appear after varying periods of time.

## POOR SITE

We use the term «poor site» when the stoma is sited in such a position as to make it difficult, if not impossible to perform the cleansing and appliance management manoeuvres, conceal the stoma under one's clothing and enjoy normal freedom of movement without fear of leakage.

Regrettably, the problem is a frequent one and, save for certain rare exceptions, bears witness to excessive haste on the part of the surgeon or a lack of cooperation with ward personnel.

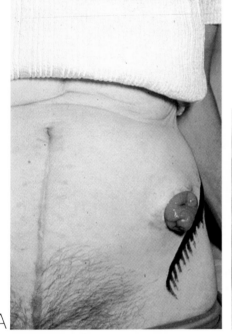

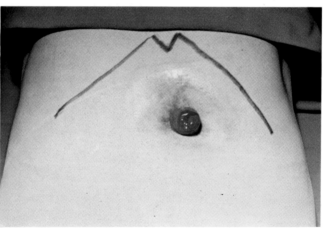

**Fig. 3.1 A, B.** A) Double-barrelled sigmoid colostomy in the region of the left iliac crest. B) Transverse colostomy close to rib cage vault.

A

B

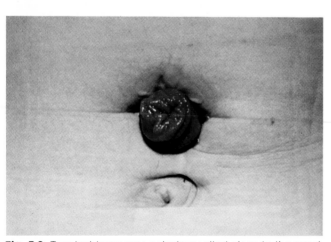

**Fig. 3.2.** Terminal transverse colostomy sited close to the navel.

The patient arrives in the operating theatre without the most appropriate site for the stoma being marked on his abdomen or the surgeon ignores any such marking or fails to comply with the basic rules when siting an improvised stoma.

Frequently, therefore, one sees stomata sited close to prominent bones (Fig. 3.1 A, B), in the vicinity of old scars or the navel (Fig. 3.2), on the main incision (Fig. 3.3) and in between folds of fat (Fig. 3.4).

Apart from concealment difficulties, awkwardness of movement and the psychological repercussions of such drawbacks, the most serious consequences of a poorly sited stoma are peristomal dermatitis and contamination of the main wound.

Should the stoma fail to be sited on a flat, smooth abdominal region, it proves very hard to get the bags to

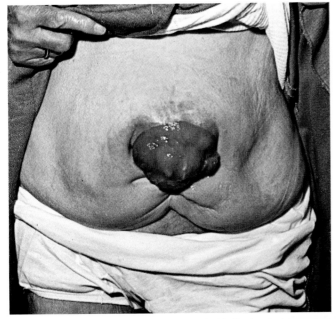

Fig. 3.3. Transverse colostomy constructed in the laparotomy area.

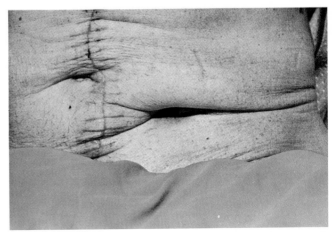

Fig. 3.4. Left terminal colostomy sited in hollow between « spare tyres ».

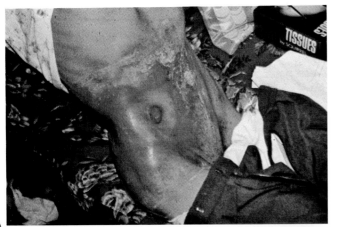

A

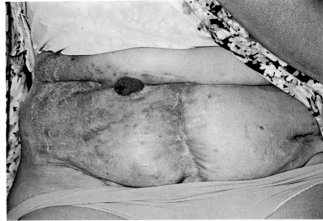

B

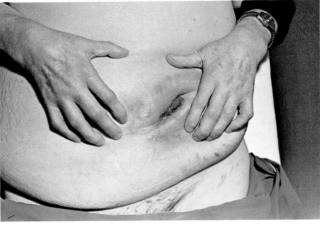

C

Fig. 3.5 A, B, C. A) Severe dermatitis of the entire right hemi-abdomen. The ileostomy is sited close to the iliac crest. B) Another example of diffuse severe dermatitis due to a poorly sited ileostomy: in this case the stoma is sited on the waist line. C) Left terminal colostomy situated in hollow between « spare tyres ». In the case of colostomy, the dermatitis is always less severe owing to the nature of the motions.

adhere perfectly with consequent leakage of faecal matter or urine and the appearance of dermatitis of varying degrees and extent (Fig. 3.5 A, B, C).

When the stoma is constructed in the main incision, there is a risk of contamination and dehiscence with consequent evisceration (Fig. 3.6 A, B).

Poor siting is therefore a serious defect even if the stoma itself is well constructed; if then, as often happens, we add a morphological defect to the faulty siting, the disturbances become intolerable and the risks are multiplied (Fig. 3.7 A, B, C), thereby necessitating by no means simple surgical operations to eliminate them.

For these reasons prevention of poor siting is of vital importance. There are general rules which it is imperative to follow (Fig. 3.8): the stoma must be sited in a flat, smooth region, far from prominent bones, i.e. the costal margins, anterior iliac spine and symphysis pu-

11

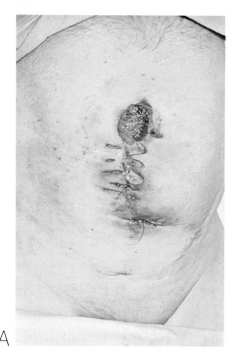

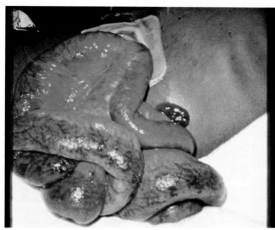

As far as siting in relation to the main incision is concerned, it must be said that the stoma should be kept out of the main incision and requires an incision of its own at an appropriate distance. This rule is so important that, if the stoma site opted for should prove to be

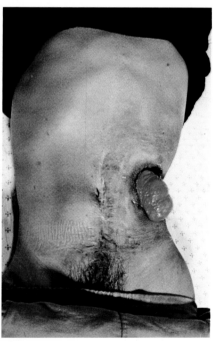

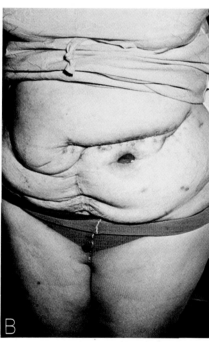

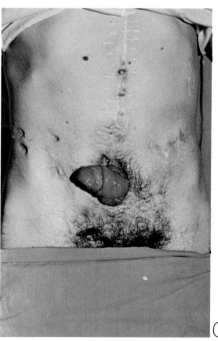

**Fig. 3.7 A, B, C.** A) Prolapsed colonic urinary conduit excessively close to the costal margin. Camouflaging with clothing is practically impossible. B) Retracted colonic urinary conduit close to the laparatomy incision. C) Prolapsed ileostomy sited on the main incision and too close to the symphysis pubis.

bis; it must be kept out of old scars; it must be located at a suitable distance from folds of fat.

Worthy of separate mention is the siting of the stoma in relation to the navel and the main incision.

As regards the former, there is a widespread view that the stoma should be sited at a distance from the navel, while some authors[73] opt for siting the stoma right on the navel, adducing as their reasons for such a location improved visibility and ease of management, especially in elderly patients.

too near the median line, a contralateral paramedian laparotomy has to be resorted to (Fig. 3.9 A, B).

In practical terms, the choice of site is conditioned by circumstances: in routine surgery the choice is made by the stomatherapist prior to the operation, taking due account of the shape of the abdomen (Fig. 3.10), the patient's life habits and the size of bag theoretically most suitable for the type of stoma planned.

It is indispensable to carry out various tests with the patient in the supine, upright and seated positions so as

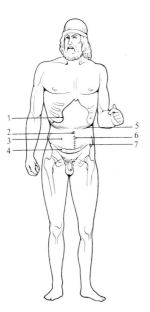

Fig. 3.8. Areas to avoid as stoma sites.

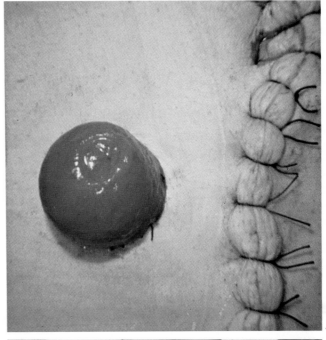

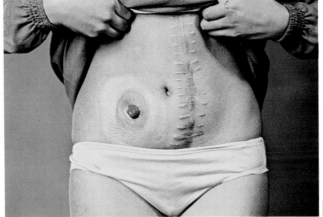

Fig. 3.9 A, B. A) Well-fashioned ileostomy, but too near the main incision. There is a risk of contamination of the wound and, in the case of cheloids, difficulty in fitting the ileostomy appliance. B) Left paramedian laparatomy to guarantee a suitable distance between main incision and stoma.

to make quite sure that the stoma is clearly visible to the patient at all times (Fig. 3.11 A, B) and does not finish up by being sited in between folds of fat (Fig. 3.12 A, B, C).

There are occasions when particular conditions of the abdomen make it necessary to locate the stoma in an usual site as in the case of a left ileostomy (Fig. 3.13).

Another exception is the siting of particular stomata such as the continent ileostomy; in such cases the traditional rules are deliberately ignored (Fig. 3.14).

If emergency surgery is necessary and there is no certainty as to the type of stoma to be constructed, it is essential for the stomatherapist to suggest several sites to the surgeon (Fig. 3.15), and this proves particularly useful in the presence of abdominal fistulas or when several drainage operations are envisaged (Fig. 3.16 A, B).

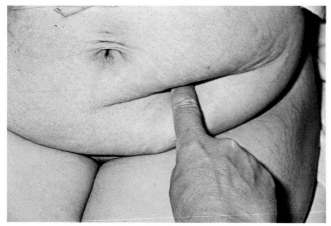

Fig. 3.10. The pre-operative examination of the abdomen of a potential ostomy patient should be extremely meticulous. Folds of fat are not always evident on simple inspection.

The stomatherapist's indications must, however, be respected at all times by the surgeon, who, for his part, will have provided the stomatherapist with adequate explanations as to the operative program; lack of co-operation may mean that unpleasant surprises are in store (Fig. 3.17 A, B).

Lastly, if the surgeon is forced to construct an improvised stoma on the spot, he should only do so in full compliance with the general rules even if the abdomen is already open and the anatomical proportions distorted. To restore normal proportions often all he need do is to bring the edges of the laparatomy wound back together temporarily with a few stitches.

A curious and entirely special situation is that of the Moslems, who prostrate themselves in prayer five times a day and must do so in conditions of perfect

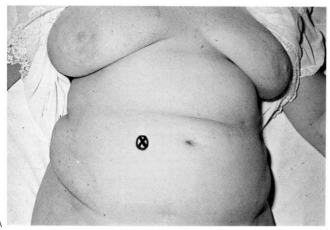

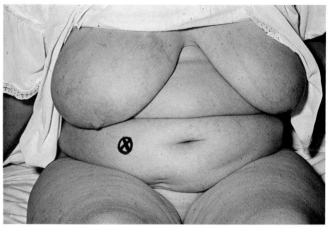

A

B

**Fig. 3.11 A, B.** The site of a transverse colostomy is marked in an obese patient in the supine position. B) The site proves satisfactory also in the sitting position: the stoma will coincide with the apex of a roll of fact and will be clearly visible to the ostomy patient.

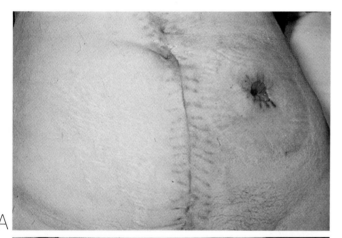

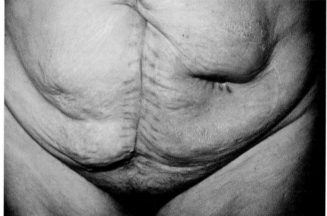

A

B

**Fig. 3.12 A, B, C.** A) Left terminal sigmoidostomy: the site of the stoma, which appeared optimal in the supine position, was not decided upon prior to surgery. B) The patient in the upright position: a fold of fat partially covers the stoma. C) The patient in the sitting position: the stoma has disappeared under the roll of fat.

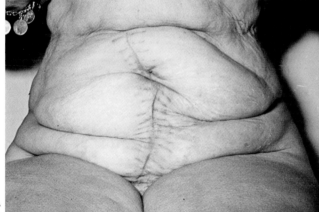

C

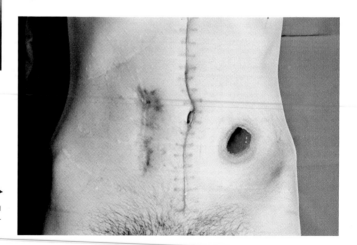

▶

**Fig. 3.13.** An ileostomy originally located in the left hemiabdomen on account of the numerous old scars present in the right quadrants.

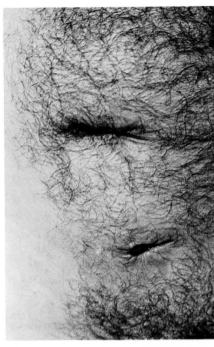

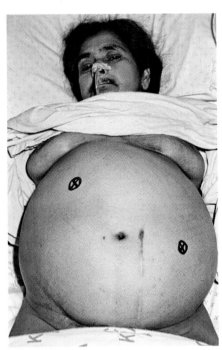

**Fig. 3.14.** Continent ileostomy: an inguinal site has deliberately been chosen, as there is no need for an ileostomy appliance and the stoma may be concealed by a minimum of clothing.

**Fig. 3.15.** Emergency surgical operation for intestinal obstruction. Suitable sites are indicated for a sigmoidostomy and a transverse colostomy, to be opted for according to necessity. In these cases the indications are approximate because the abdominal distension distorts the normal anatomical proportions.

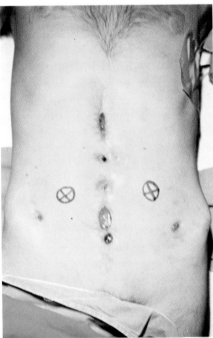

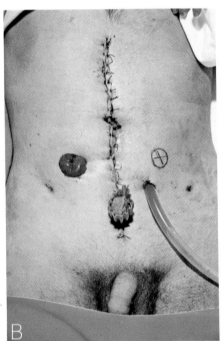

**Fig. 3.16 A, B.** A) Patient operated on several times for Crohn's disease of the ileum. On this occasion a colectomy was planned together with an ileostomy. Two possible sites were indicated for the stoma in view of the fact that the presence of numerous fistulas and the likely need for several drainage operations made it impossible to draw up a precise plan. B) It proved possible to construct the stoma in the traditional site.

**Fig. 3.17 A, B.** An example of what can happen if co-operation between surgeon and stomatherapist is lacking. In a patient operated on several times for Crohn's disease (A) the surgeon performs an atypical incision so as to simplify access to the abdominal cavity and concludes the operation by siting a colostomy (B) in the region of the curvilinear incision and close to the left iliac crest.

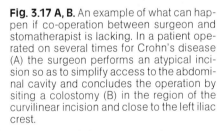

A

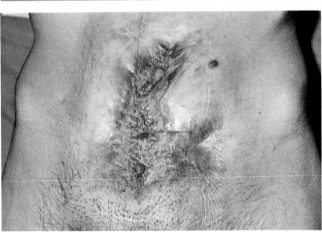

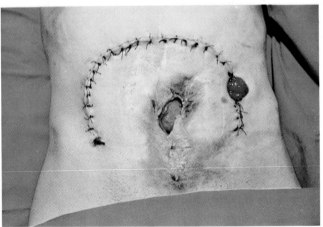

B

cleanliness of the body below the navel. If a Moslem has to have a stoma, it must therefore be sited above the navel to prevent the passing of motions during genuflexion from annulling the benefits of prayer (Fig. 3.18).

As regards the remedies for a poorly sited stoma, it should be said that, at least in terminal colostomies, mechanical regulation of the bowel by irrigation makes it possible to obviate the main problems by freeing the patient from the slavery of colostomy bags (Fig. 3.19).

With the other types of stomata the only effective measure is to re-site the stoma, as all alternative remedies, including the most elaborate and ingenious discharge collection systems, prove ineffective or too complicated in relation to the manual or intellective capabilities of many ostomy patients.

The surgical operation consists in closing the original stoma and opening another in an appropriate site, which, of course, is identified prior to surgery and is often located in the contralateral hemiabdomen (Fig.

3.20 A, B). Generally speaking, the same bowel segment is used, but in some cases it proves necessary to change not only the site but also the type of stoma (Fig. 3.21).

The operation is intricate and involves the re-opening of the main incision, difficulties of access to the peritoneal cavity and laborious mobilization manoeuvres to guide the stomal loop to its new site. For this reason the operation is justified only if the patient is suffering severe hardship and is indicated only if the stoma is of the permanent type and there is no longer any trace of the original disease.

## OEDEMA

Stomal oedema may constitute a pathological manifestation in its own right, may complicate other pathological events such as stenosis and prolapse or, lastly, may be deemed physiological in the course of natural occurrences such as pregnancy.

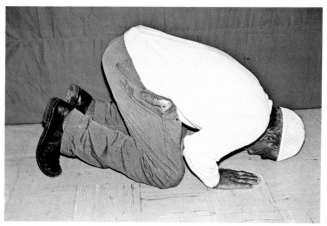

**Fig. 3.18.** Moslem at prayer; the stoma has to be sited above the navel for religious reasons.

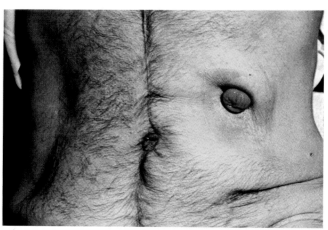

**Fig. 3.19.** A left terminal colostomy sited close to the lower costal margin. The colostomy appliance cannot be fitted, but the use of irrigation makes it possible to do without the colostomy bag.

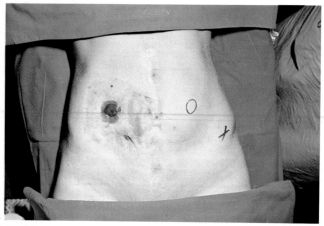

A

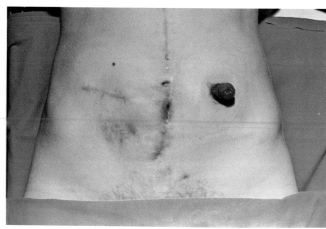

B

**Fig. 3.20 A, B.** A) Ileostomy sited at the centre of an area devastated by surgical scars and fistulas. As a result of serious management problems the stoma must be re-sited in the left quadrant. B) The new stoma proves perfectly manageable.

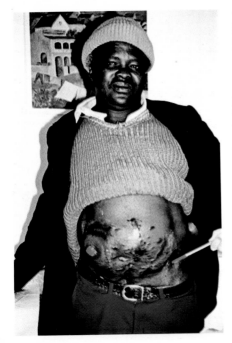

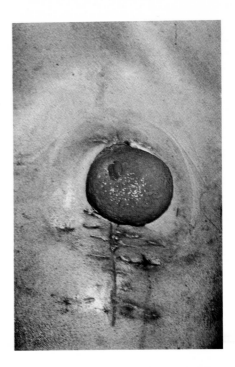

**Fig. 3.21.** A resited transverse colostomy replacing a sigmoid loop colostomy sited low in the left groin.

**Fig. 3.22.** Oedematous transverse colostomy due to cutaneous stenosis. In this case, a further factor contributing to the oedema is faecal stagnation due to inadequate opening of the bowel.

In this section we shall examine only the first condition, in which the oedema is due to on obstructed venous discharge caused by extra- or intraluminal factors.

In the extraluminal case the oedema sets in acutely, is manifested in the immediate postoperative period and is generally of marked degree: the stoma appears to be of abnormal size, swollen, turgid and taut (Fig. 3.22).

In the intraluminal case, which is much rarer, the oedema sets in surreptitiously, progresses slowly and is at no time conspicuous; the stomal mucosa tends to take on a pale, atrophic aspect (Fig. 3.23).

The most common extraluminal causes are inadequacy of the parietal opening in relation to the size of the exteriorized bowel (Fig. 3.24 A, B) and pressure exerted by the support rod beneath a poorly mobilized loop (Fig. 3.25). Among the most frequent intraluminal causes we have relapse of the original disease and stagnation of faecal matter.

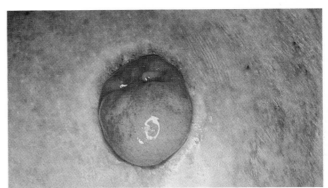

**Fig. 3.23.** Oedema due to intraluminal causes in a terminal sigmoidostomy. The mucosa is pale and atrophic.

**Fig. 3.24 A, B.** A) Oedematous ileocaecal loop conduit due to stenosis of the parietal aperture. B) The same with the appliance attached.

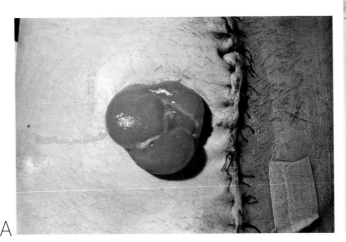

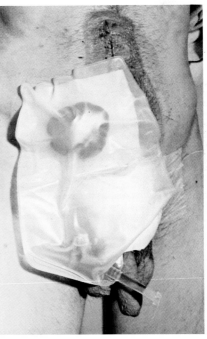

A

B

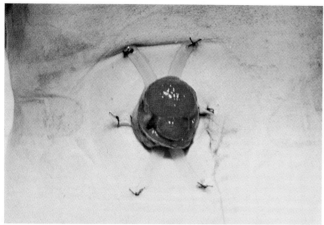

**Fig. 3.25.** Oedematous transverse colostomy due to compression of the rod in a poorly mobilized portion of bowel.

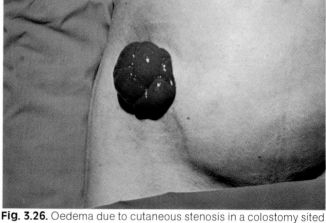

**Fig. 3.26.** Oedema due to cutaneous stenosis in a colostomy sited close to the iliac crest. The oedema prevents discharge of the faeces and the patient's stoma remains occluded.

From the subjective point of view the patient may experience pain at the first passage of motions, but, above all, he is alarmed at the sight of a stoma which is much greater in size than he had imagined.

In the case of chronic oedema the progressive change in the stomal morphology seriously alarms him and prompts him to seek the surgeon's help.

In functional terms the oedema, according to its degree of severity, may have negative effects ranging from partial discharge difficulties to complete obstruction (Fig. 3.26). The phenomenon is more frequent in colostomies, given the greater degree of solidity of the faecal matter, but it may also occur in ileostomies with a particular mechanism: in the presence of a conspicuous oedema the faecal matter stagnates, increases in density as a result of an excess of water resorption and not only contributes towards maintaining the oedema but actually even aggravates it. In ileal and colonic urinary diversions the oedema may give rise, albeit rarely, to a stoppage of urine emission with very serious consequences, even to the extent of causing hydronephrosis (Fig. 3.27 A, B, C).

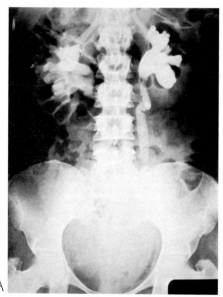

A

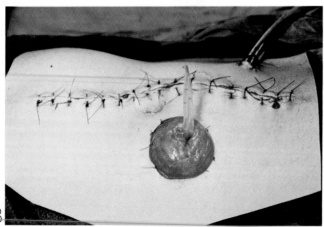

B

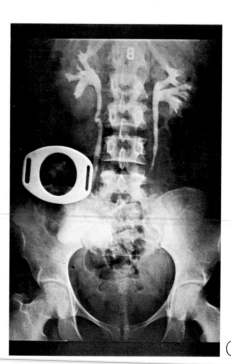

C

**Fig. 3.27 A, B, C.** Acute ureteric dilatation (A) caused by obstruction due to stomal oedema in an ileal loop conduit despite the use of ureteric stints (B). Once the oedema has been resolved, the urinary output is normalized and the ureteric dilatation reduced (C).

Acute postoperative oedema usually regresses spontaneously as soon as the obstacle to venous discharge, for instance the support rod, is removed.

Oedema due to a disproportion between the bowel diameter and the parietal aperture also tends to regress by virtue of physiological accomodation phenomena. In those rare cases where this does not happen the stoma will need to be corrected surgically by slightly broadening the parietal aperture, even under local anaesthetic, at the skin or fascial level according to the location of the stenosis.

In the case of chronic oedema, on the other hand, the therapeutic problem is bound up with the treatment for recurrence of the original disease.

Stomal oedema, therefore, does not usually pose the surgeon major problems, and it is his task, above all, to prevent it by making an adequate parietal incision and by ensuring a sufficient degree of bowel mobilization. On the stomatherapist's part, on the other hand, it calls for painstaking assistance based upon affording the ostomy patient the necessary psychological support and upon regular monitoring of the stomal function.

We have already mentioned the psychological aspect: the more assurances the ostomy patient has received that his stoma will be small in size, the greater will be his disappointment and disheartenment.

He needs to be reassured that the phenomenon is temporary and can be put right with relatively simple expedients. The monitoring of stomal function takes the form of continual supervision of the patient. If the abdomen is distended and the emission of faecal material scanty, one should first delicately explore the stoma and then proceed with the fluidification of the bowel contents by instilling small quantities of lukewarm water (Fig. 3.28 A, B).

Lastly, as regards stoma management, it is essential to take due account of the dimensions of an oedematous stoma, and therefore appliances of appropriate size must be resorted to. In addition, it is good practice to use two-piece appliances so as to facilitate frequent inspection of the stoma without damaging the skin.

## ISCHAEMIA

Ischaemia appears early on and may involve the entire stomal loop or an extensive portion of it, in which case we refer to it as total ischaemia, or it may be confined to the exteriorized portion and is thus defined as partial or terminal ischaemia. The former situation is due to a vascular lesion caused during the mobilization manoeuvres or, more frequently, in the peritoneization phase when the mesentery of the stomal loop is used to close the paracolic gutter. Devascularization, then, may occur as a result of section of an artery or ligation (Fig. 3.29).

As early as the first few hours after surgery the entire stoma is already in the throes of ischaemic necrosis (Fig. 3.30).

A delicate exploration reveals the extent of the phenomenon within the stomal loop and suggests the need for an immediate re-operation consisting in the resec-

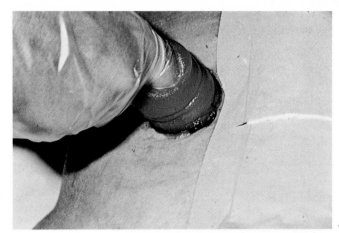

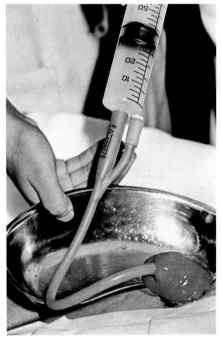

**Fig. 3.28 A, B.** A) Digital exploration of an oedematous ileostomy. B) Insertion of a catheter into the stoma and delicate instillation of warm water so as to soften the faecal mass or obstructive bolus.

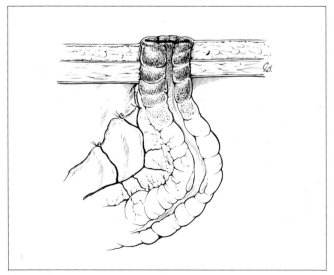

**Fig. 3.29.** Diagram illustrating the pathogenesis of ischaemia.

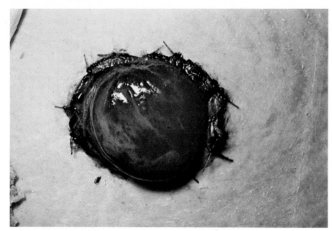

**Fig. 3.30**. Total necrosis due to ischaemia.

tion of the necrotic part and the construction of a new stoma.

This situation can be avoided by a meticulous intraoperative check on the vascularization: if the surgeon is not absolutely sure of the vitality of the loop joining the abdominal wall, he has no choice but to wait as long as is necessary for the situation to become quite clear, and, should the situation fail to improve as

the minutes pass or, indeed, tend to deteriorate, he should not hesitate to eliminate the distressed loop.

Partial ischaemia may be due to compression exerted on the bowel by the edges of an excessively narrow parietal opening, to tension caused by insufficient mobilization or, lastly, to excessive skeletization of the terminal portion of the stomal loop.

In the first two cases the vascular damage is almost always of a venous nature and consists in haematic infarction which rapidly causes the stoma to turn cyanotic and oedematous without, however, any sign of necrosis. The phenomenon, which is generally transient and tends to clear up spontaneously, rarely requires surgical measures such as the refashioning of the parietal incision under local anaesthetic.

In the third case, however, the vascular damage is arterial in origin and occurs when there is extensive devascularization beyond the 3-4 distal centimetres of the stomal loop, as is done to assist the eversion of the mucosa or to facilitate the mucocutaneous suture, in conjunction with a relatively insufficient vascularization of the submucosa.

The stoma rapidly manifests signs of ischaemic necrosis, which, however, is of a sectorial nature (Fig. 3.31 A, B, C, D).

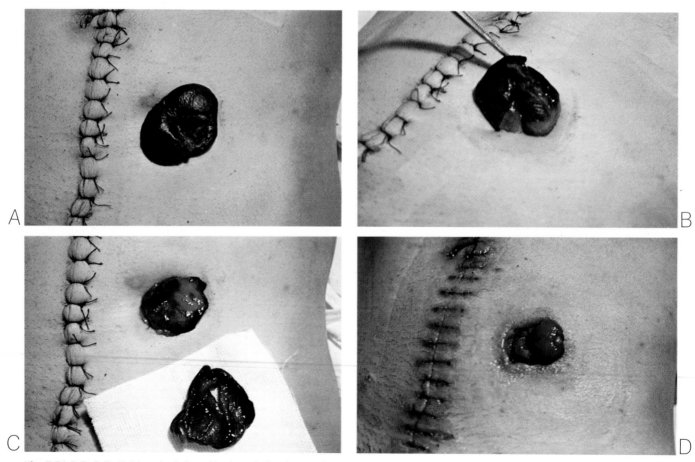

**Fig. 3.31 A, B, C, D.** A) A terminal sigmoidostomy in the throes of ischaemic necrosis. B) Inspection reveals that the ischaemia is of the partial type. C) Removal of the portion of necrotic bowel. Areas of residual necrosis and well-vascularized areas are clearly visible on the stoma. D) After a few days the stomal mucosa appears well-vascularized, though slightly oedematous. There is a thoroughly cleansed partial mucocutaneous detachment.

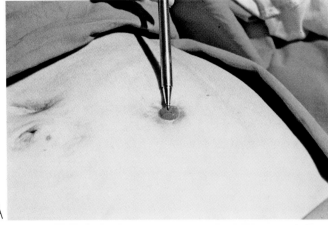

A

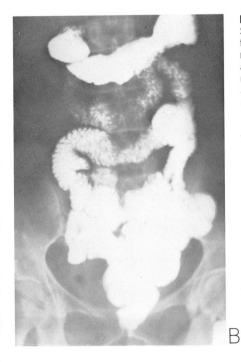

**Fig. 3.58 A, B, C.** A) Stenosis of a left terminal colostomy constructed as a result of a Hartmann sigmoid resection for neoplasm. B) In an examination per os of the alimentary tract the colon is not visualized since the entire ileal content passes into the ampulla via an ileorectal fistula. C) Canalization occurs via the natural route. The dermatitis is due to the continual leakage of ileal contents from the anus.

B

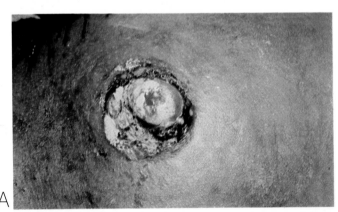

C

Early stenoses, due to the disproportion between the diameter of the bowel and that of the parietal incision, appear together with the stomal oedema.

Late stenoses, which are asymptomatic in the initial phases, always finish up by causing ingravescent disturbances as the stoma progressively shrinks in diameter and grows increasingly rigid (Fig. 3.60 A, B, C).

Apart from the now rare cases of ileostomy dysfunction already mentioned above, stenosis in colostomies gives rise to substantial discharge difficulties with consequent faecal stagnation and abdominal tension as well as hyperfermentation or faecal putrefaction phenomena. To all this we should add the pain experienced on passing solid matter, not to mention the difficulties involved in irrigation manoeuvres or in performing trans-stomal diagnostic investigations by such

◄

**Fig. 3.59 A, B, C.** Phosphate collections due to stenotic urinary diversions with subsequent alkaline and infected urine: A) a large cutaneal urostomy, B) an ileal conduit, C) a flush colonic conduit.

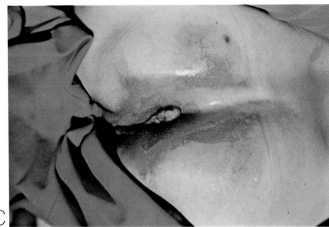

A

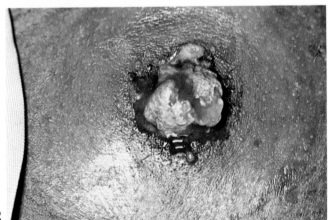

B

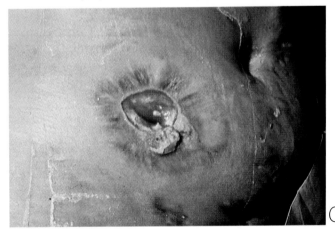

C

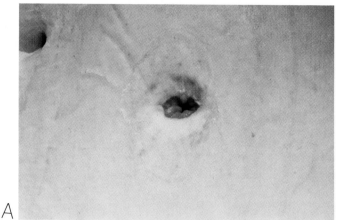

A

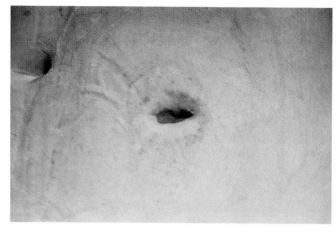

B

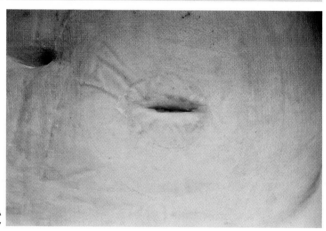

C

**Fig. 3.60 A, B, C.** A) Progressive stricture of a terminal colostomy. In this phase the stenosis is practically asymptomatic. B) The diameter has narrowed and discharge difficulties are setting in. C) The stoma has become a rigid fissure. The evacuation difficulties are now considerable. It is impossible to perform irrigation.

peristomally. To avoid a relapse the operation must necessarily be completed with a new mucocutaneous suture.

It is essential to ensure perfect haemostasis, otherwise the resulting peristomal haematoma could be infected and suppurate, thereby laying the foundations for a relapse.

## PROLAPSE

Prolapse consists in the excessive protrusion of the stomal loop out of the abdominal skin.

Although there are some authors who use the term «prolapse» only in those cases where the protrusion exceeds 6 centimetres,[16] it is more correct to consider as prolapsed any stoma which protrudes more than it

methods as the barium enema or, above all, endoscopy.

From the therapeutic point of view conservative measures are largely inefficacious and are justified only if the ostomy patient's general conditions are compromised.

Digital and instrumental dilatation may, if anything, slow down the process and may be resorted to, at best, only in the initial phases (Fig. 3.61).

When the disturbances increase, there is no alternative but to correct the stenosis surgically, and this may be done by minor operations, occasionally under local anaesthetic.

If the stenosis affects only the skin rim, a circular peristomal incision is performed at a distance of a few millimetres from the mucosal margin. The terminal portion of the loop is resected slightly below the skin ring and a new mucocutaneous suture is performed (Fig. 3.62 A, B, C, D, E, F).

If the stenosis is at fascial level, all that is necessary is an incision in the aponeurosis just sufficient to ensure a congruent aperture.

In these cases, it is wise to clamp the apex of the fascial incision with a stitch so as to obviate the risk of a subsequent vibex and thus a peristomal hernia.

If, lastly, the fibrosis affects the entire transparietal cylinder, all the newly formed tissue must be removed

**Fig. 3.61.** Instrumental dilatation of a stenotic left colostomy.

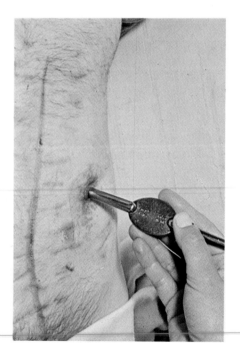

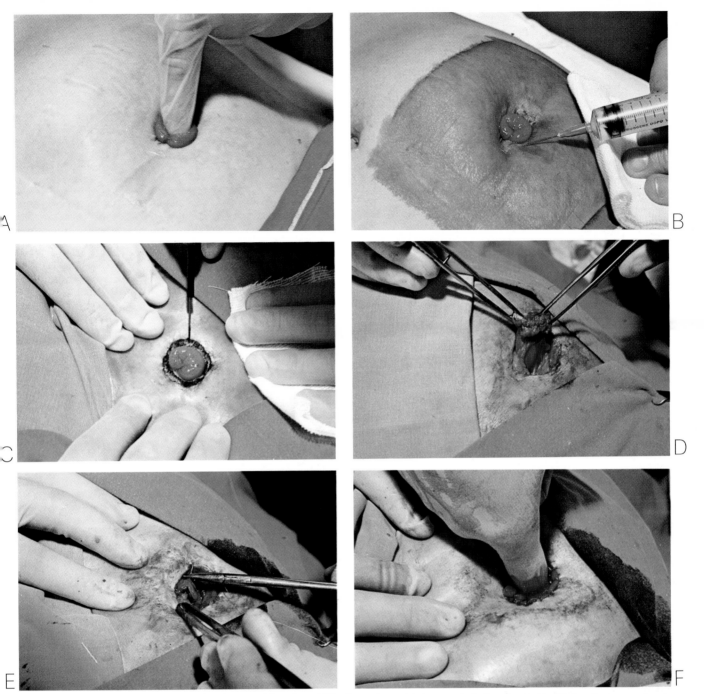

**Fig. 3.62 A, B, C, D, E, F.** A) Stenotic left colostomy. The gloved little finger is unable to penetrate the rim of skin. B) Surgical correction is performed under local anaesthetic. C) Circular skin incision at a distance of a few millimetres from the mucosal edge. D) The terminal portion of the colon is removed. E) Completion of the new mucocutaneous suture. F) The stoma is now soft and broad in diameter. It affords ease of access on the part of the gloved index finger.

did at the time it was constructed. The prolapse concept, in fact, implies an idea of progression and thus length should be considered as a variable attribute, which can be used to indicate the proportions of a prolapsed stoma but not as an element in its definition.

We distinguish between a mucosal prolapse and a total prolapse. The former, comparable to the prolapse in the rectum, consists in the sliding of the mucosa on the muscular tunics which remain fixed, while, in total pro-

lapse, which resembles intussusception, the entire bowel cylinder slides on itself, the fixed point in this case being the mucocutaneous margin.

A mucosal prolapse never assumes proportions of more than 3-4 centimetres. Total prolapse, on the other hand, may prove to be of very substantial dimensions (Fig. 3.63).

All stomata are potentially subject to prolapse, but the phenomenon is markedly more frequent in colos-

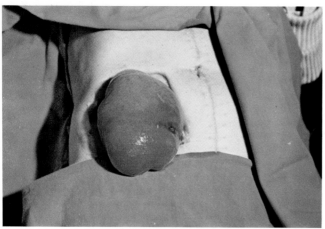

**Fig. 3.63.** Enormous colostomy prolapse. The portion of exteriorized bowel extends from the waist line to the groin and occupies almost all the right hemiabdomen.

tomies, especially those of the double-barrelled «loop» type. Allington Jr.,[5] in 1892, considered it inevitable and defined it as a disagreeable drawback which the patient needed to be informed about.

Of all stomal pathological manifestations, prolapse is the most frequent, with percentages ranging from 20 to 50%[13,45,76] and afflicts up to 14% of ostomy patients.[16]

In double-barrelled loop colostomies, prolapse of the distal loop should probably be considered the more frequent,[16] but not all authors take this view,[45] and in effect it is reasonable to assume that the possibilities actually break even (Fig. 3.64 A, B, C).

From the aetiological point of view, we should distinguish between predisposing factors and actual causes. Among the former, once we have dealt with the influence of the patient's sex and the original disease, which would not appear to affect prolapse at all, we have to take into account the patient's age, in the sense that prolapse is much more frequent in children than in adults, the type of stoma, whether terminal or double-barrelled, and its localization in terms of the

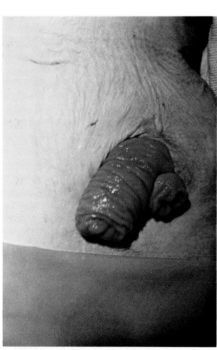

A

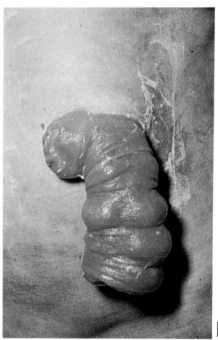

B

**Fig. 3.64 A, B, C.** A) Double-barrelled sigmoidostomy: prolapse prevalently of the proximal loop. B) Transverse loop colostomy: prolapse of the distal loop. C) Double-barrelled sigmoidostomy: prolapse of both loops with exteriorization of the spur.

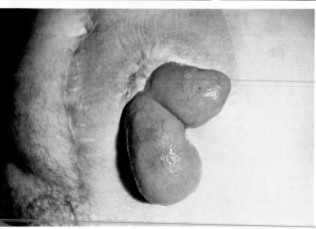

C

portion of colon used; the more proximal portions on the whole tend to be more subject to prolapse, at least in adults.

Another relevant factor consists in obstructions of the distal colon. Colostomies constructed for an obstructive disease of the colon prolapse more easily than others, with a ratio of more than 5 to 1.[16]

The explanation of this phenomenon is to be found in the disproportion between the stomal incision, judged to be appropriate at the time surgery took place, and the new dimensions which the colon takes on once it is decompressed.

Peristalsis and all conditions which increase endoabdominal pressure have an effect on the growth of the

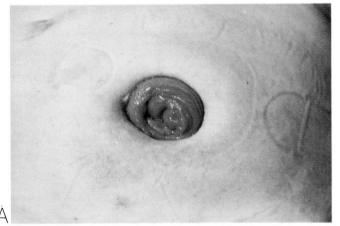
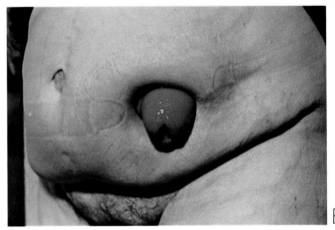

A                                      B

**Fig. 3.65 A, B.** A) Excessively wide stomal incision. B) Predictably, the stoma is prolapsed.

prolapse, once it has set in, rather than on its actual genesis.

For all these factors to be able to exert their influence, there has to be an existing structural defect in the stoma. This concept, which has long been considered fundamental, has recently been questioned but cannot be refuted.

The most common defects are: excessive width of the stomal incision (Fig. 3.65 A, B), summary preparation of the bowel to be exteriorized, as when too much omentum is left on the transverse colon, and, above all, inadequate visceroparietal fixation. By the latter we mean both inadequate anchorage of the bowel to the fascia and an inadequate suture of the mesentery to the parietal peritoneum of the paracolic gutter (Fig. 3.66).

From the clinical point of view the main problems arising from the prolapse relate to stomal hygiene and containment of faecal matter (Fig. 3.67 A, B). To these we should add the problems relating to camouflaging or concealment in the very bulky forms. The prolapse, in fact, though hardly ever irreducible, is always uncontainable and appears spontaneously in the erect position; it is, therefore, not easy for the patient to conceal it under his clothing, especially when, for example, in an emotional state peristaltic waves are generated which alter the proportions and shape of the prolapsed stoma (Fig. 3.68 A, B).

Another problem is bleeding. The size of the prolapsed loop, in fact, favours minor traumatisms responsible for erosion and ulcerations of the mucosa which are liable to bleed. The blood collects in the bag, mingling with the faeces, and alarms the patient, who immediately associates it with a recurrence of the original disease (Fig. 3.69).

Strangulation is a rare occurrence and is generally put right by means of the reduction manoeuvre. The latter, at times, may prove very laborious, but ostomy patients are usually capable of performing it on their own, and emergency admissions to hospital are not frequent in relation to the incidence of prolapse.

In such cases one has to resort to the application of ice and hypertonic solution compresses.

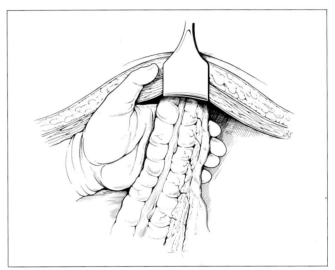

**Fig. 3.66.** One of the technical conditions responsible for the formation of the prolapse: the mesosigmoid is not anchored to the internal abdominal wall and the bowel slides freely on itself.

The reduction manoeuvre should be performed with considerable caution by gently squeezing the oedematous bowel, out of which ooze large amounts of serohaematic liquid. An attempt is then made to reduce it, working with both hands, starting from the distal portion, and progressively making sure that the portion of bowel eased back into the abdomen does not slide out again, protruding as before (Fig. 3.70 A, B, C).

Strangulation may occur in a rigid ring appliance, and, in this case, after patient squeezing, the bag support must be cut through and removed (Fig. 3.71).

The consequences of strangulation are bowel obstruction and ischaemia.

The former hardly ever has time to transform itself into actual occlusion because the reduction of the prolapse is usually done promptly. The phenomenon is more serious when it occurs in a prolapsed urostomy owing to the risk of urinary stagnation with consequent hydronephrosis and sepsis. In such cases, even before

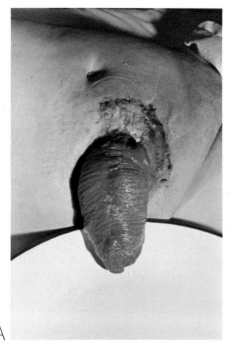

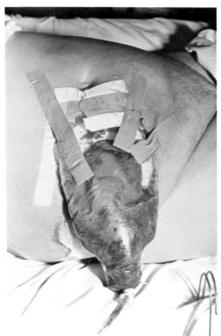

**Fig. 3.67 A, B.** A) Voluminous colostomy prolapse with protrusion of the ileocaecal valve. In such conditions great difficulties arise with regard to stomal hygiene. B) Continence and management also become harassing problems. This patient was bed-ridden and used complicated contrivances involving sticking plaster and a collection tube attached with elastic bands to the bottom of the bag.

A

B

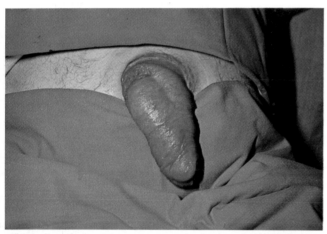

A

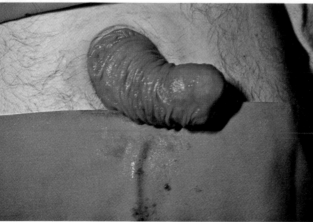

B

**Fig. 3.69.** In prolapses of large proportions bleeding is fairly frequent. Blood mingling with the faeces is visible through the appliance.

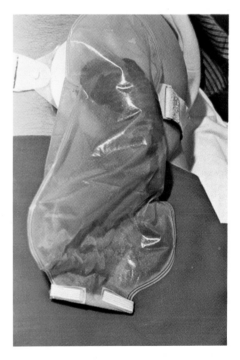

**Fig. 3.68 A, B.** A) Enormous prolapse of transverse colostomy, difficult to conceal owing to its position and bulk. B) Spontaneous contraction of the prolapsed bowel with substantial alteration of shape, position, volume and consistency. Variations of such proportions are detectable to the naked eye even when covered by clothing.

attempting the reduction manoeuvre, a catheter must be introduced into the stoma in order to relieve the pressure on the neovesica (Fig. 3.72 A, B).

Ischaemia, too, generally does not have time to bring about necrotic phenomena. The reduction manoeuvre should be very delicate on account of the fragility of the portion of bowel in the throes of vascular distress (Fig. 3.73 A, B).

From the therapeutic point of view, conservative treatment offers few chances of success: the ostomy

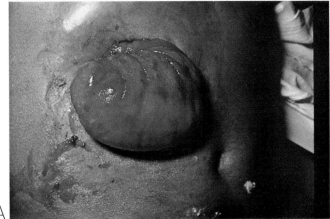

A

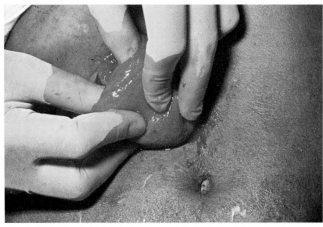

B

**Fig. 3.70 A, B, C.** A) Strangulation of a prolapsed transverse colostomy. The stoma appears turgid, hyperaemic and oedematous. B) The reduction manoeuvres are performed delicately using both hands to squeeze the bowel and progressively force it back in. C) The prolapse has been temporarily reduced.

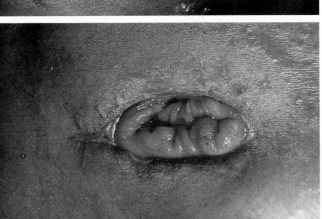

C

**Fig. 3.72 A, B.** A) Strangulation of a prolapsed colonic urinary diversion. A probe is delicately introduced in order to relieve the pressure on the neovesica. B) With the neovesica emptied the prolapse can be reduced.

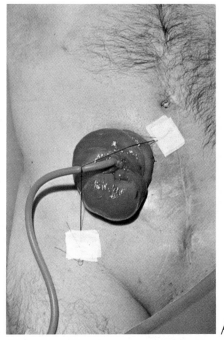

A

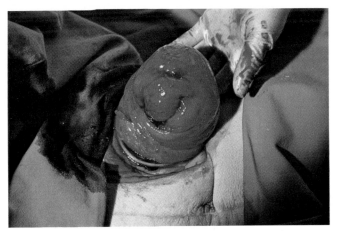

**Fig. 3.71.** Strangulation of a colostomy prolapse. The cause of the stricture is the plastic ring of the colostomy appliance.

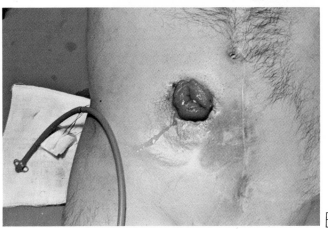

B

patient can be taught to reduce the prolapse before fitting the stoma appliance. Stoma bags with rigid or semirigid supports must be ruled out as these favour strangulation. A management system has to be devised which takes account of the conformation of the abdomen, the type of stoma and the size of the prolapse.

As regards surgery, the choice lies between a vast range of possible operations. As in the case of many other pathological stomal manifestations, the type of

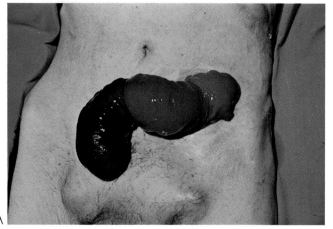
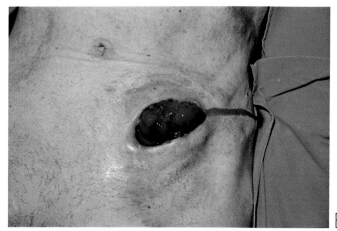

A

B

**Fig. 3.73 A, B.** A) Enormous prolapse of a double-barrelled sigmoidostomy in the strangulation phase. The ischaemic distress of the terminal portion of one of the loops is clearly visible. B) In such cases the reduction manoeuvres must be performed with extreme delicacy and great care. The trickle of sero-haematic fluid is produced by the squeezing of the bowel.

surgery indicated depends upon the extent of the disturbances, the general condition of the ostomy patient and the nature of the stoma itself. If the stoma is temporary and the prolapse very troublesome, this could be sufficient reason for anticipating the date of surgery.

We distinguish between minor operations which are confined to eliminating the prolapse disturbances without tackling the cause and major operations which involve a laparotomy and are aimed at solving the problem from an aetiological point of view.

Among the former we should mention button colopexy, a technique recently brought to surgeons' attention[99] (Fig. 3.74 A, B).

Another method consists in the mucoparietal anchorage of the bowel by means of a purse-string suture (Fig. 3.75 A, B, C, D, E, F).

The most rational procedure, however, is decapitation of the prolapse (Fig. 3.76 A, B, C).

In all three cases, the surgical measures involved are simple, reasonably efficacious and, in any case, useful as means of alleviating distressing situations.

The major surgical operations involve a laparotomy and consist in performing a fresh, tenacious fixation of the stomal loop by firmly anchoring its mesentery to the internal part of the abdomen or in the reconstruction of the stoma in a new site (Fig. 3.77 A, B, C, D).

These are operations which offer absolute guarantees but which are indicated only in terminal-type stomata and in subjects in good general shape.

## PERISTOMAL HERNIA

This consists in an unmistakeable yielding of the abdominal wall due to complete or partial detachment of the aponeurotic fascia from the stomal loop (Fig. 3.78 A, B). The contents of the hernia, usually consisting of the loops of the small intestine with their parietal peritoneum lining, make their way through this aperture, spreading into the subcutaneous region and creating for themselves the space they require (Fig. 3.79 A, B).

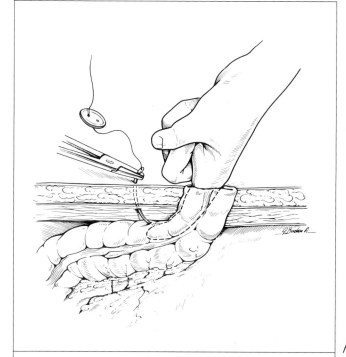

A

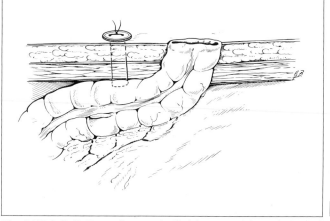

B

**Fig. 3.74 A, B.** Button colopexy. A stitch is passed through the wall and the surgeon attempts to get hold of the loop using his finger as a guide.

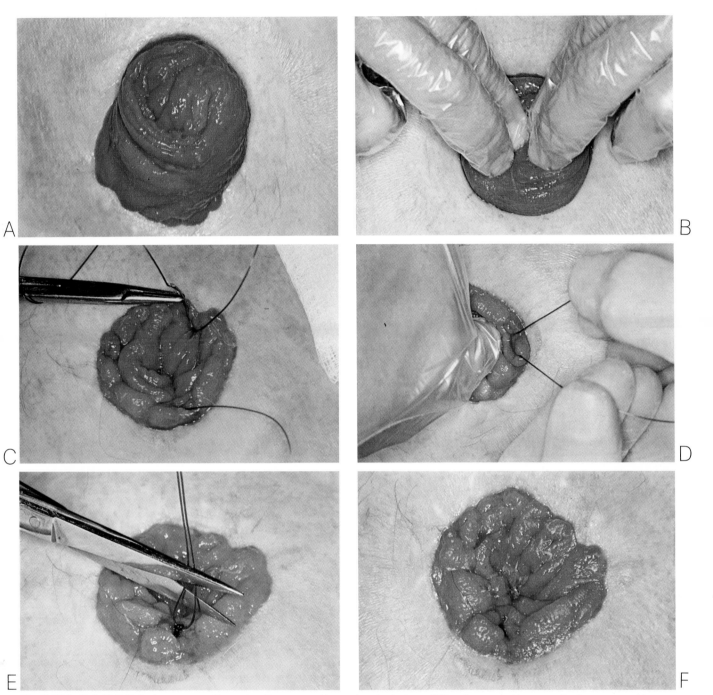

**Fig. 3.75 A, B, C, D, E, F.** Prolapse correction using the purse-string suture technique. Without any need for anaesthetic, a purse-string suture is performed by passing a non-absorbable stitch from the mucosa into the peristomal subcutaneous tissue and taking care each time to re-insert the needle in the same hole from which it has just emerged. On completion of the purse-string suture around the entire stomal circumference, the knot is tied, at the same time measuring the stoma diameter with a finger, and the thread is cut. Care should be taken to bury the knot between the mucosal folds below skin level.

Peristomal hernias vary very considerably in size and sometimes assume huge proportions (Fig. 3.80).

There is no preference for sex or age, although in elderly patients the yielding of the tissues tends to be more frequent and more complete.

Herniation may occur in any type of stoma but is rare in ileostomies, which are usually constructed in young patients and function without any increase in abdominal pressure (Fig. 3.81). As regards colostomies, frequencies of more than 7% are to be found in literature,[43, 76] whereas hernia frequency in ileostomies is less than 2%.[36]

Peristomal hernia is almost always due to a technical error committed during construction of the stoma.

The most common defect is making an excessively wide fascial incision, i.e. more than 2-3 centimetres in diameter.

An empirical, yet none the less valid method of avoiding this error consists in gauging the incision with the fingers and making sure that it is barely large

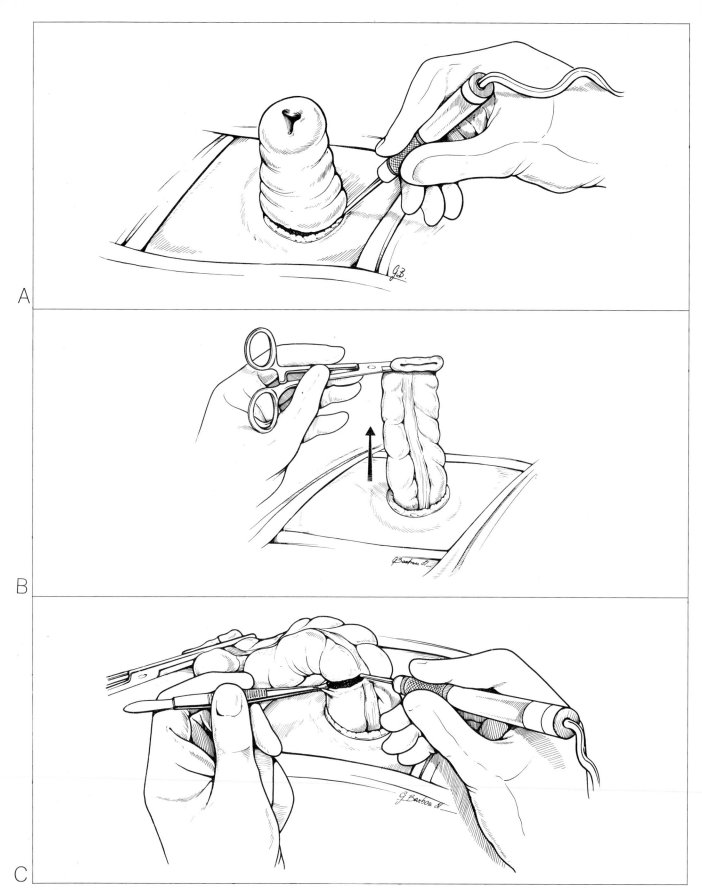

**Fig. 3.76 A, B, C.** Decapitation of the prolapse. This can be performed under local anaesthetic and consists in the amputation of the portion of prolapsed bowel. The mucosa is detached from the skin, the loop is drawn out and transected at a suitable point allowing the surgeon to refashion a new eversion or perform a flat mucocutaneous suture according to whether he is dealing with an ileostomy or, as illustrated here, a colostomy.

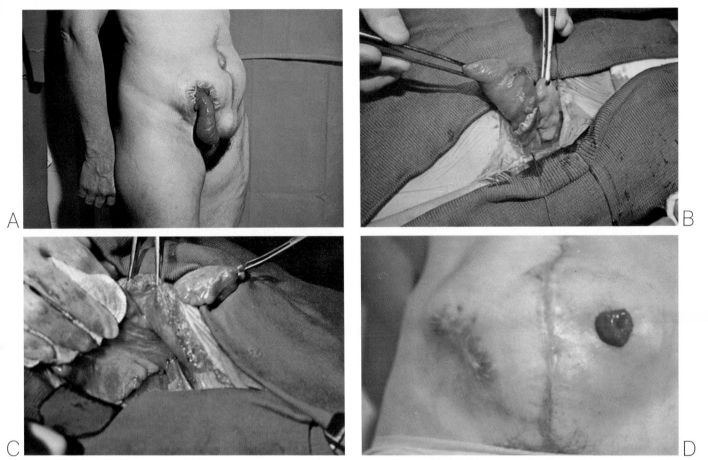

**Fig. 3.77 A, B, C, D.** A) Correction of the prolapse by means of the stoma re-siting method, in this case an ileostomy. B) Detachment of the stoma. The slide illustrates the pathogenesis of the stoma; nothing prevents the free ileal loop from continuing to slide into the prolapsed cylinder thereby increasing its length. C) The ileum is brought to the skin via a fresh incision cut in the left hemiabdomen. The mesentery of the stomal loop hangs in festoons on the promotory of the sacrum to which it must be firmly anchored if relapse is to be avoided.

enough to take the forefinger and middle finger together. If the incision is narrower than this, there is a risk of stenosis; if it is broader, it ought to be reduced with a stitch or two, otherwise herniation is guaranteed to take place and will set in early.

**Fig. 3.78 A, B.** A) Peristomal hernia in the site of a terminal sigmoid colostomy with detachment of the aponeurosis around the entire circumference of the stomal loop. B) Peristomal hernia in the site of a left colostomy with aponeurotic detachment confined to the lower semicircumference.

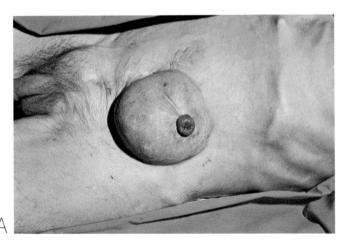

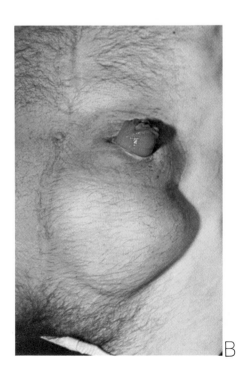

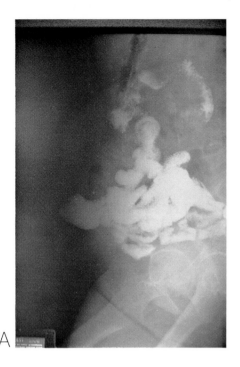

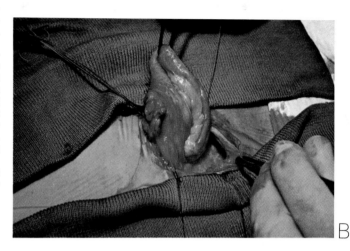

**Fig. 3.79 A, B.** A) Radiogram of the alimentary tract showing the presence of a loop of the small bowel beyond the shadow area of the abdominal wall. This loop constitutes the contents of a peristomal hernia. B) In this intraoperative slide, the same loop as in the radiogram can be seen adhering to the colon, which is closed by a purse-string suture. Also visible is the subcutaneous cavity into which the loop was insinuating itself.

A

B

ing of the fascial defect and forcing the abdominal contents between the stomal loop and the fascial edge.

The diagnosis of peristomal hernia is reached by inspection and palpation and is, in any event, a simple matter, provided you ask the patient to strain and cough as is normal practice in diagnosing any type of

Another causative factor is an unsuitable site, as when the stoma lies outside the rectus muscle, for instance in the region of the groin, in the lateral quadrants or at the apex of the main laparotomy wound.

A further cause is the progressive yielding of the aponeurosis, as may occur in elderly patients, even if the original incision was of the right size and the surgeon, in such cases, was actually not to blame.

Clearly any condition, such as obesity, constipation, prostatism or coughing, which tends to produce an increase in endoabdominal pressure may accelerate and aggravate the process contributing towards a broaden-

hernia. As a rule, tumefaction appears as soon as the patient assumes the erect position; in the more voluminous cases, the hernia presents as a more or less regular dome-shaped bulge with the stoma aperture at its summit; the actual stoma is not necessarily altered.

Subjectively, herniation is the source of three distinct types of disturbances, which may be more or less severe and, acting either alone or all together, finish up by becoming intolerable: psychological distress, abdominal alterations and impeded stoma management.

The herniary swelling is unaesthetic and is very difficult to conceal under the clothing (Fig. 3.82 A, B, C,

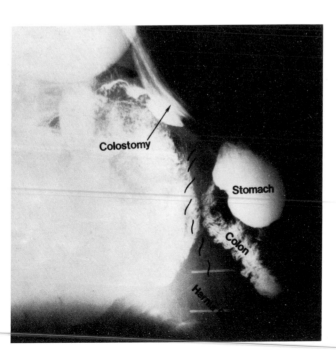

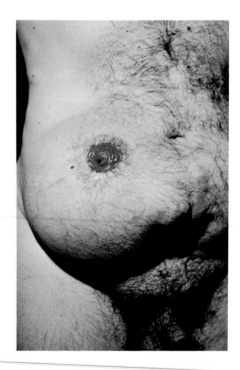

◀

**Fig. 3.80.** Peristomal hernia of giant proportions. In this slide taken in profile, the radiological examination of the alimentary tract shows most of the stomach and the transverse colon which have slipped into the hernia sac.

▶

**Fig. 3.81.** A rare example of a hernia in the site of an ileostomy, which in this case is also retracted.

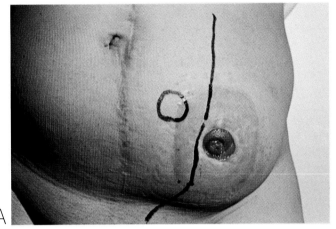

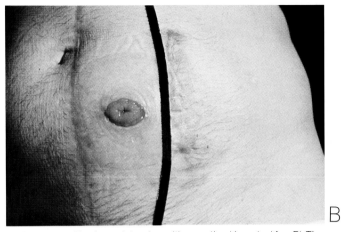

A

B

**Fig. 3.89 A, B.** A) Peristomal hernia in the site of a low, laterally sited sigmoidostomy. The homolateral re-siting method is opted for. B) The new stoma is again in the left hemiabdomen and the incision has been made in the region of the rectus muscle.

**Fig. 3.90 A, B, C, D, E.** A) Peristomal hernia in the site of a sigmoid colostomy.. The method adopted is homolateral re-siting with implantation of the magnetic ring. B) The old stoma is completely detached and protected; the hernia sac is opened and resected. The new disc incision is made on the same side but higher up than the previous incision. C) Frontal insertion of the magnetic ring. D) The new stoma is complete, as is the aponeurotic plastic surgery of the old incision. All that remains is to close the skin wound. E) End result.

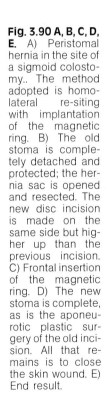

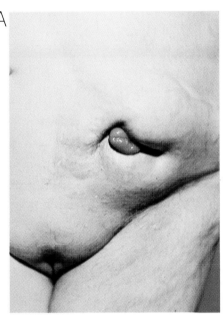

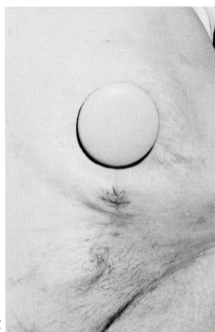

A

E

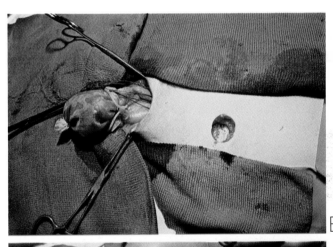

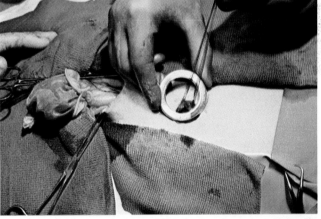

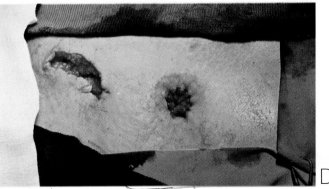

B

C

D

the prevention of a recurrence (Fig. 3.90 A, B, C, D, E).

In point of fact, even if there are authors who claim that the ring is of no use in preventing hernia,[47] it cannot be denied that the intrusion of bowel between the loop and the ring is highly unlikely, if not impossible, just as it seems extremely hypothetical that the aponeurosis may yield at a distance from the stomal loop, i.e. beyond the circumference of the ring.

Whatever the method opted for, the surgical tehcnique needs to be meticulous. The operation must not fail to achieve its objective, because a recurrence of hernia is very embarrassing not only for the surgeon but also for the ostomy patient himself, who is no longer prepared to tempt fate and finds himself obliged to put up with his disturbances.

## GRANULOMAS

The term «granuloma» is commonly used to describe all those productive formations of a benign nature which appear on the surface of the stoma, even through many of these are not actually granulomas in the strict sense of the term.

This group of lesions comprises granulomas due to foreign bodies, aspecific fibroproductive nodules and inflammatory pseudopolyps.

Foreign-body granulomas are the common granulomas caused by sutures and are generally located on the mucocutaneous edge either in a single sector or along the entire circumference (Fig. 3.91). They are often accompanied by peristomal fistulas, with which they have in common the same aetiological aspect which can be traced back to phlogosis caused by visceroparietal fixation stitches (Fig. 3.92).

The fibroproductive nodules are also located on the mucocutaneous edge, but usually affect only the lower semicircumference. They are entirely aspecific, made up, as they are, of chronic inflammatory tissue with the characteristics of productive fibrosis, and represent the reaction of the edge of the stoma to the chronic trauma brought about by the stoma appliance (Fig. 3.93). They

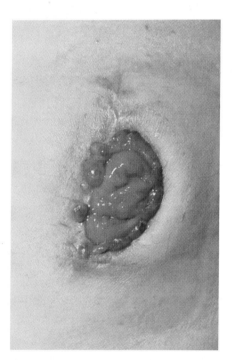

**Fig. 3.91.** Granulomas due to foreign body around the circumference of a double-barrelled sigmoidostomy.

**Fig. 3.92.** Stitch granuloma and peristomal fistula at the base of an ileostomy.

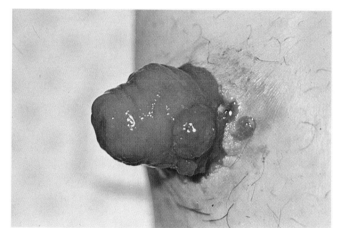

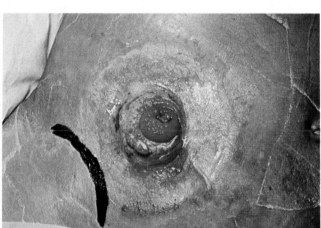

**Fig. 3.93.** Fibroproductive reaction on the edge of a poorly sited ileostomy close to the ileac crest. To avoid infiltration of faecal matter, the patient used a rigid appliance which he held pressed against his abdomen by means of a very tight belt.

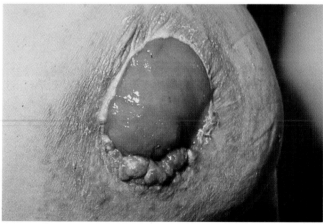

**Fig. 3.94.** Fibroproductive nodules on the lower semicircumference of a colostomy. The stoma is misaligned and its orifice points downward giving rise to continual contact between the faeces and the bottom edge of the stoma.

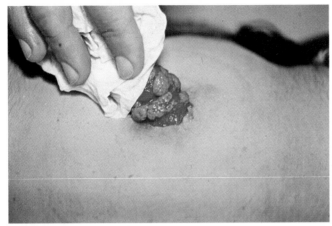

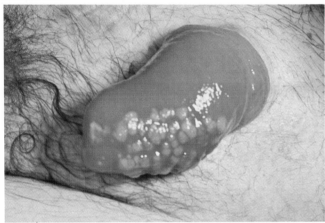

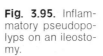

Fig. 3.95. Inflammatory pseudopolyps on an ileostomy.
◄

Fig. 3.96. The term «inflammatory pseudopolyp» is due to the contemporary presence of newly formed granulation tissue, visible at the centre of the photograph, and of hyperplastic glandular formations in the muciparous depletion phase.
►

Fig. 3.97. Inflammatory pseudopolyps on a prolapsed colostomy.
◄

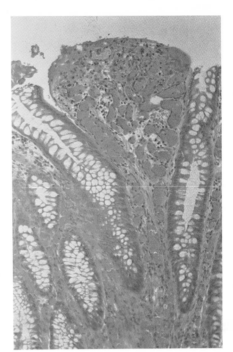

are very frequent in misaligned stomata, in which the orifice points downwards and the motions come into contact with only one sector of the stomal circumference (Fig. 3.94).

Lastly, we have the inflammatory pseudopolyps, which are confined to the stomal mucosa and do not affect the mucocutaneous edge (Fig. 3.95).

The name is due to the fact that they prove to be made up not only of granulation tissue but also of hyperplastic granular tissue starting out from the mucosa (Fig. 3.96).

Like fibrous nodules, inflammatory pseudopolyps, too, are due to chronic trauma brought about by rigid stoma appliances and are aided and abetted by the existence of other pathological stomal manifestations, particularly prolapse (Fig. 3.97).

The diagnosis presents no difficulties and is based on simple inspection, except in the case of those patients operated on for Crohn's disease, where a biopsy should be performed to exclude the possibility of a recurrence on the stoma.

With regard to the disturbances the patient experiences, those caused by inflammatory pseudopolyps are generally only slight; more troublesome are the lesions of the mucocutaneous edge which give rise to pain and a burning sensation on passing motions.

As far as treatment is concerned, apart from correction of the original stomal defect, which is the basic predisposing factor, other remedial measures to be taken consist in the adoption of soft, well-fitting stoma appliances and cauterizing with silver nitrate (Fig. 3.98 A, B) or electro-diathermy (Fig. 3.99 A, B, C).

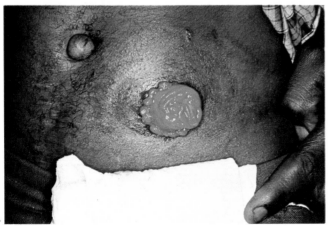

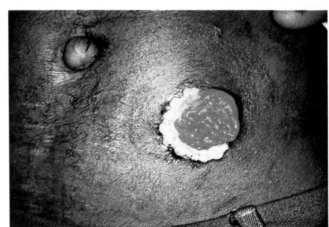

A                                                                                                      B

Fig. 3.98 A, B. A) Suture granulomas around a sigmoid. B) Caustication of the granulomas with silver nitrate.

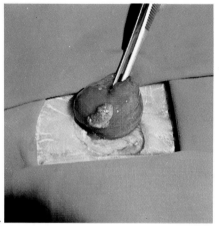
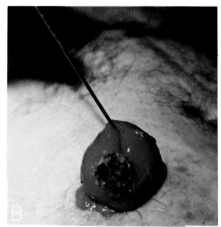
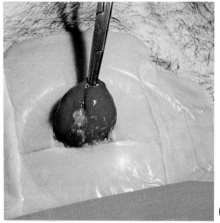

A                                                                                        B                                                                                        C

**Fig. 3.99 A, B, C.** A) Inflammatory pseudopolyp on an ileostomy. B) The cauterization has been performed using electro-cautery. C) In a few days the loss of substance has been made up.

## TRAUMAS

The ostomy patient is just as subject to abdominal traumas as anyone else, especially now that progress in rehabilitation techniques has enabled him to lead a normal life.

The stoma may thus be involved in traumas due to road accidents, sporting mishaps or physical aggression and as a result may suffer all kinds of lesions ranging from contusion to laceration.

These are complex situations which are not easy to classify and cannot be accommodated in any rigid scheme of treatment. The type of surgery, where necessary, is chosen in the field not only in relation to the actual damage suffered by the stoma but also in relation to damage suffered by other portions of intestines. It is not always possible to conserve the original stoma and, indeed, it may often prove necessary to replace it with another in a new site.

In any event, these situations fall within the domain of general traumatology and must be considered as abdominal traumas in an ostomy patient.

Stomal traumas in the strict sense of the term are those which are directly related to stoma management practices and manoeuvres and may be classified as internal and external, depending upon where the lesion occurs, and as acute or chronic, depending upon the mechanism of action of the agent responsible for the lesion.

The most common *internal stomal trauma* is perforation of the stomal loop occurring in the course of irrigation or a barium enema, the agent responsible for the lesion in such cases being a probe or catheter which is either excessively rigid or is introduced without due care.[83] Perforation may be considered a somewhat rare occurrence, if we bear in mind that the cases reported in literature are of the order of a hundred or so, counting both those occurring during wash-out and those caused by a barium enema.[56]

Factors predisposing towards perforation include pre-existing pathological stomal manifestations such as hernia, stenosis or prolapse and particular situations such as alcoholism, psychic disturbances and inexperience due to inadequate instruction, which lead to improper manoeuvres on the patient's part.

Another factor is the presence of disease of the stomal loop, particularly diverticulosis (Fig. 3.100).

The perforation may be intraperitoneal, intramesenteric or extraperitoneal.[56] Of these, intraperitoneal perforation is the most common and occurs somewhere along the stomal loop in a position proximal to its transparietal portion at a variable distance from the stomal orifice (Fig. 3.101).

The clinical picture is that of diffuse peritonitis, all the more serious the greater the quantity of liquid which collects in the peritoneum. The prognosis is unfavourable unless treatment is prompt and radical.

Intramesenteric perforation is rare; the lesion occurs on the mesenteric edge of the loop at a variable distance from the stoma (Fig. 3.102).

**Fig. 3.100.** Intraperitoneal perforation in the course of irrigation. The lesion is visible immediately below the stoma and the lozenge of skin removed. Two errors should be emphasized in this case: the stoma was constructed on a diseased colon (diverticulosis) and irrigation was recommended to an ostomy patient with such a colonic condition.

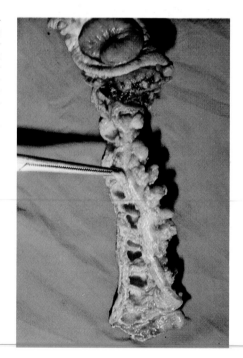

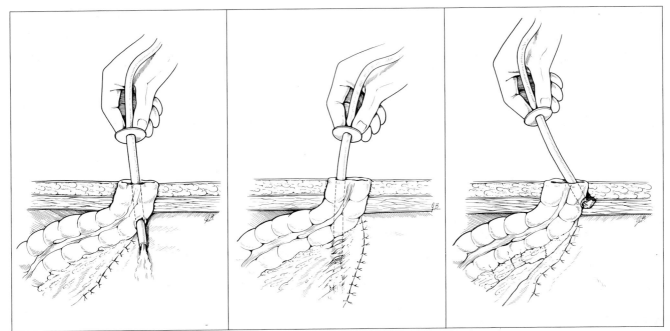

**Fig. 3.101.** Intraperitoneal perforation caused by irrigation cannula.

**Fig. 3.102.** Intramesocolic perforation caused by irrigation cannula.

**Fig. 3.103.** Intraparietal perforation caused by irrigation cannula.

The symptoms set in surreptitiously but take on dramatic form as soon as the intramesocolic abscess, which forms immediately, gives rise to the necrosis of the stomal loop.

The prognosis is very grave even despite radical treatment.

Extraperitoneal perforation occurs along the transparietal portion of the stomal loop and manifests itself in the form of an abscess in the abdominal wall (Fig. 3.103). The treatment consists in draining off the fluid which has collected.

*External stomal traumas,* i.e. those affecting the bowel segment protruding above skin level, may be acute or chronic and can appear in any type of stoma.

Acute external traumas are fairly frequent but of only minor significance in terms of their consequences. Generally speaking, these are superficial mucosal lesions due to imprudent cleansing manoeuvres or clumsy attempts to reduce a prolapse, occasionally prompted by fits of anger on the part of the ostomy patient or a desire to inflict self-injury.

These lesions give rise to haemorrhages which may even be very intense, often alarming the patient and inducing him to seek hospital assistance. These haemorrhages do not present treatment problems and tend to clear up spontaneously.

Episodes of this kind, however, should put the stomatherapist on the alert because they invariably imply a regression on the ostomy patient's part as regards his ability to manage his stoma or an exacerbated state of psychological distress.

Chronic traumas, which are also very frequent, are due to the repeated action of rigid stoma appliances or

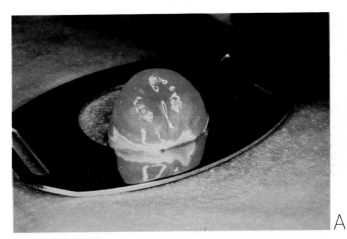

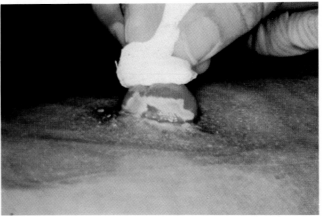

**Fig. 3.104 A, B.** A) Chronic trauma at the base of an ileal loop diversion. The agent responsible for the lesion is a metal stoma faceplate. B) The lesion presents the characteristics of a transverse fissure in the cicatricial fibrosis phase.

51

parts of such appliances on the mucosa of the exteriorized bowel loop.

Such traumas occasion productive lesions, inflammatory pseudopolyps or losses of substance, represented, on the one hand, by trans-stomal fistulas and, on the other, by a series of polymorphous lesions including erosions, fissurations and ulcerations.

Inflammatory pseudopolyps and fistulas have already been dealt with in separate sections above. Polymorphous lesions are commonly observable, especially in ostomy patients who over a period of years fail to present themselves for periodic check-ups in hospital or stomatherapy centres. It thus comes about that these patients, who have long deprived themselves of up-to-date information and are unaware of new developments, continue to use antiquated appliances of the type in use at the time they were operated on, i.e. appliances fitted with rigid supports, occasionally even metal ones (Fig. 3.104 A, B).

Such appliances, in continuous contact with the exteriorized mucosa, cause lesions which do not get a chance to heal properly through normal re-epithelization on account of the constant repetition of the trauma.

The lesions may be confined to a single sector of the stoma or may affect its entire circumference (Fig. 3.105).

In the initial phase, the predominant symptom is bleeding; in the course of time, a fibrous reaction of a cicatricial type sets in, which, in transverse fissurations, may lead to stomal stenosis.

The treatment of such lesions is conservative; it consists in immediately adopting a soft stoma appliance and in protecting the stomal mucosal edge with natural protective pastes (Fig. 3.106).

## SKIN LESIONS *

The peristomal skin is subject to pathological alterations associated with operative trauma, contact with faecal and liquid discharge and the use of stoma appliances.

These forms of dermatitis were undoubtedly more frequent in the past owing to the greater number of defective stomata, the use of less refined materials in the stoma appliances and the habit of using irritating substances to cleanse the stoma, but even to-day they are by no means rare.

### Dermatitis due to trauma

These forms of dermatitis may be due to operative trauma or to the damaging action of stoma appliances.

To understand dermatitis due to operative trauma, we should first recall a number of the basic general concepts of dermatology.

It is a known fact that apparently healthy skin areas

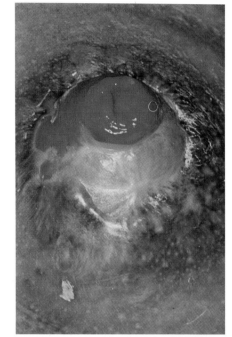

**Fig. 3.105.** Serious chronic trauma in an ileal loop conduit due to rigid stoma appliance. The stoma has lost the tunica mucosa around its entire circumference. The bleeding, fibrotic submucosa is visible.

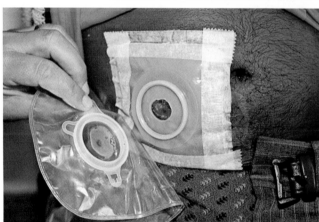

**Fig. 3.106.** The same case as in Fig. 3.105. The metal faceplate has been replaced by a much softer one. The use of a two-piece appliance makes it easier to keep a frequent check on the lesion and simplifies local treatment.

in a patient suffering from certain forms of dermatosis, if subjected even to very slight traumas such as a pin-prick, may reproduce the basic dermatosis at the point stimulated.

This phenomenon, whose essential mechanism has never actually been explained, is termed an isomorphic reaction (Behçet's disease, pyoderma gangrenosum) or, to use eponyms, Nikolsky's sign (pemphigus) or Koebner's sign (psoriasis, lichen ruber planus).

Behçet's disease, an aphthosis of the oral and genital mucosae with hypopion and relapsing iritis, is characterized by the occurrence of nodular papulopustular lesions which may reproduce themselves in the sites of even the very slightest traumatism.

Pyoderma gangrenosum, which is often associated with ulcerative colitis and a serious immunological deficit, consists in lesions of an ulceronecrotic, sero-pus-secreting type with a chronic relapsing trend. These le-

* By Professor A. MONTAGNANI, Director of the Dermatological Clinic of the University of Bologna.

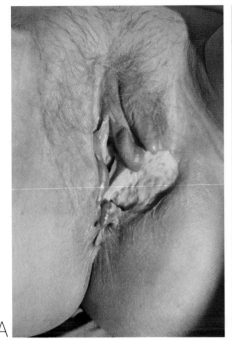

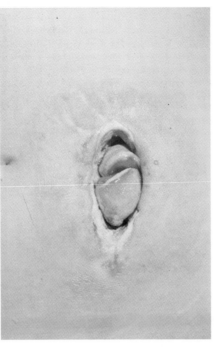

A

B

**Fig. 3.107 A, B.** A) Pyoderma gangrenosum of the perineal region with vulvar and anal involvement. B) Peristomal isomorphic lesion caused by surgical trauma.

sions may reproduce themselves in a trauma site, for instance, on a cutaneous stomal incision (Fig. 3.107 A, B).

Pemphigus, particularly in the chronic bullous variety, but also in chronic pemphigus vegetans and pemphigus foliaceus, counts among its pathognomonic symptoms the reproduction of blisters or epidermal peeling phenomena on healthy skin due even to very mild traumatisms (Nikolsky's sign).

In psoriasis, a chronic relapsing disease characterized by erythemato-squamous lesions, and in lichen ruber planus, whose typical manifestations are shiny, pruriginous papules, the sign of isomorphic reaction (Koebner's sign) occurs with the appearance of erythemato-squamous patches or the formation of papules respectively in a trauma site (Fig. 3.108 A, B).

It is clear that in the presence of one of these diseases the surgeon should bear in mind the possibility that an isomorphic lesion will appear in the site of the stoma incision.

In the case of psoriasis, this risk remains indefinitely, whereas in the case of pyoderma gangrenosum the skin reactivity may disappear with the healing of the primitive focus (Fig. 3.109 A, B, C).

Isomorphic reactions must be differentiated from sores due to the stoma appliance, which resemble those of the gums, cheeks or tongue as a result of the use of dentures and consist in losses of substance of varying depth which cause pain and heal quickly when the type of appliance is changed.

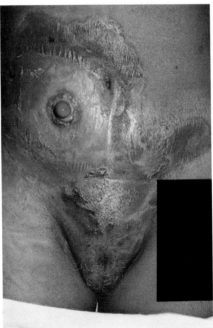

**Fig. 3.108 A, B.** In a patient suffering from psoriasis (A), surgical trauma has triggered off an intense isomorphic reaction (B).

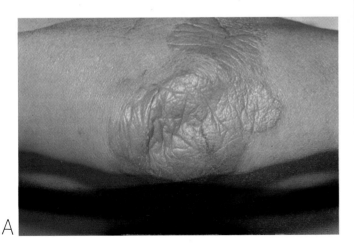

A

B

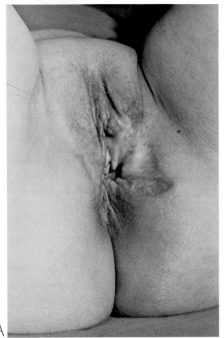
A
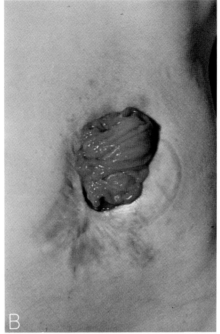
B
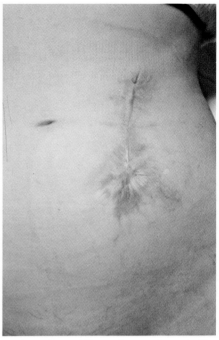
C

**Fig. 3.109 A, B, C.** The same case as in Fig. 3.107. In gangrenous pyoderma the healing of the primary focus (A) may be accompanied by the regression of the isomorphic lesion (B) and by the disappearance of the cutaneous reactivity so that the closure of the stoma occurs without any aftermath (C).

## Contact dermatitis

The discharge of faecal matter and effluent liquids from the stoma and the secretions of the everted mucosa continuously moisten the skin and may macerate it (Fig. 3.110), causing the upper surface layers of the epidermis to peel off, thereby preparing the skin itself for dermatitis due to contact with the substances of which the stoma appliance is made.

Eudermia, or good functionality of the skin, depends not only upon the integrity of its structures (epidermis, dermis, subcutis) and adnexa (pilosebaceous complexes) but even more upon the degree of protection afforded the skin by morphofunctional and biophysical components.

These are the horny layer consisting of keratinized epithelial cells (keratin, by its very nature, is extremely resistant both to acidic substances and even very powerful alkaline substances) and the hydrolipidic mantle or anaderma, composed of the sudosebaceous mixture which endows the surface of the skin with its impermeability and with a neutral or slightly acidic pH, capable, for its part, of maintaining the resident cutaneous flora in a saprophytic condition.

The use of alkalizing or cleaning substances (soaps, disinfectants, non-anionic cleansing agents) on the skin, i.e. substances capable of eliminating the hydrolipidic mantle and modifying the surface pH, and the persistence on the skin of liquid or semiliquid matter (liquid discharge, faeces, sweat) with consequent maceration of the horny layer, are conditions which alter the equilibrium proper to eudermia and thereby expose the skin to aggression on the part of external fac-

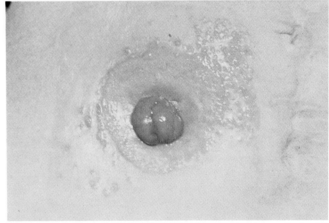

**Fig. 3.110.** Maceration of the peristomal skin due to contact with faecal discharge.

tors both of an infectious nature (germs and fungi) and of a chemical nature (antigens, haptenes).

We must distinguish, then, between dermatitis of an infectious nature and dermatitis caused by chemical attack.

The forms of dermatitis belonging to the former type may be caused by both germs (staphylococci and pyogenic streptococci) and fungi or yeasts of the *Candida albicans* genus.

The pyogenic germs may give rise to eruptions both of the intertrigo type (erythematous spots with the presence of seropurulent exudation) and of the bullous impetigo type (eruption of vesico-blisters with seropurulent contents on normal or erythematous skin).

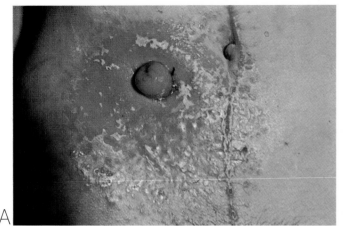

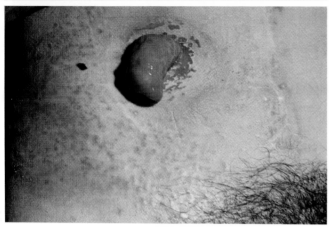

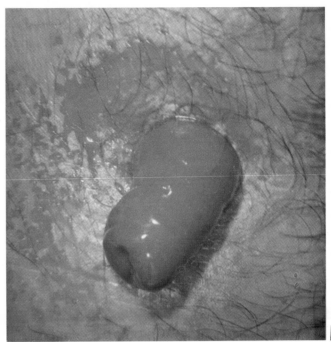

**Fig. 3.111 A, B, C.** Three examples of peristomal candidiasis.

*Candida albicans* establishes itself and multiplies on moist, macerated skin, making it go intensely red and shiny, and gives rise to the formation of a white-coloured or dirty-white adherent film (Fig. 3.111 A, B, C).

The forms of dermatitis due to chemical attack, also called eczematous contact dermatites, constitute the most frequent peristomal skin reactions.

In patients with a predisposition towards dermatitis either because they are atopic or on account of previous sensitizations due to drugs, cosmetics, clothing, jewelry, work materials, etc. and with the peristomal skin prepared by maceration caused by liquid discharge, faeces, sweat or the use of cleansing agents, contact with the substances of which the stoma appliance is made may give rise to a reactive dermatitis.

The materials most commonly used in the stoma appliances are polyethylene, acrylic resins, rubber, adhesive substances and, in the case of the more recent appliances, also natural resins, carboxymethylcellulose, amides, etc.

All these substances and their components may sensitize the skin or act as haptenes on skin which is already sensitized, and it is thus possible that contact between the stoma appliance and the skin – particularly skin already prepared by the effects of traumas, macerations and skin cleaning – will give rise to a form of contact dermatitis which, at least in the initial stages, reproduces the size and shape of the actual contact (Fig. 3.112 A, B, C).

The symptoms are classic: the dermatitis is preceded and accompanied by itching, a bright red erythema appears (Fig. 3.113 A, B, C) which may be flat or stand out in relief due to oedema (erysipeloid), and is then followed by vesiculation (Fig. 3.114 A, B) and serum secretion.

These symptoms persist as long as the contact lasts and may complicate as a result of the onset of concurrent pyogenic (impetiginization) or mycotic forms (candidiasis).

The healing of dermatitis takes place after a scale-scab phase (Fig. 3.115) perhaps with temporary hyperpigmentation (Fig. 3.116), whereas the chronic phase (Fig. 3.117 A, B) is entered into with a thickening of the skin which turns slate-grey in colour, accompanied by accentuation of the skin furrows and folds and a possible increase in the horny layer or so-called lichenization (Fig. 3.118).

Once contact dermatitis has set in, it does not tend to heal unless the cause is removed. As, however, the patient cannot do without a stoma appliance, it becomes imperative to prevent the formation of dermatitis.

To this end it is necessary to take a very thorough case history so as to identify previous history of eczema or contact dermatitis due to cleansing agents, metals, paint, drugs, cosmetics, etc.

If a previous history of this type is discovered, epicutaneous tests must be performed with the substances making up the stoma appliances; in the choice of stoma apliance to be used even those with only one positive-tested component must be ruled out.

In addition, it is absolutely essential to take the maximum possible care in constructing the stoma so as to

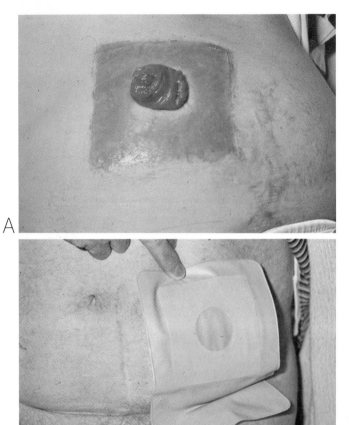

A

B

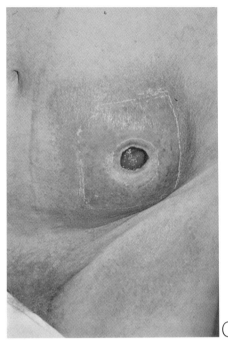

C

**Fig. 3.112 A, B, C.** Contact dermatitis reproduces the shape and size of the actual contact. It may be caused only by a part of the appliance, generally the adhesive flange (A) or by the entire bag (B and C).

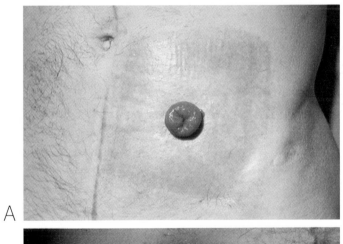

A

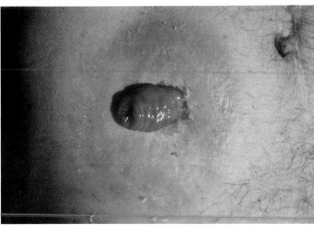

B

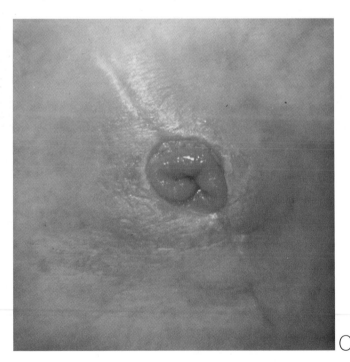

C

**Fig. 3.113 A, B, C.** Three examples of pruriginous erythema, the initial phase of dermatitis due to chemical attack.

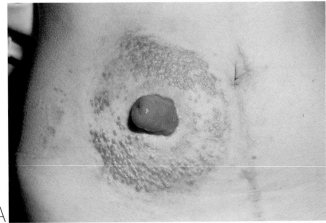

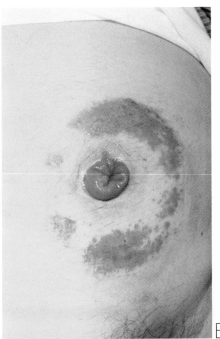

**Fig. 3.114 A, B.** Second phase of dermatitis due to chemical attack with the formation of blisters with serous (A) or haemorrhagic content (B).

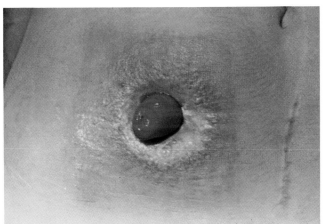

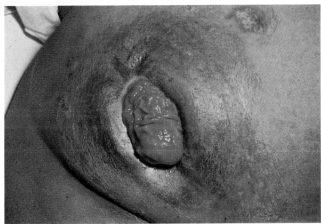

**Fig. 3.115.** Scale-scab phase in the healing of peristomal dermatitis due to chemical attack.

**Fig. 3.116.** Hyperpigmentation concludes the healing process in dermatitis due to chemical attack and is visible even in a coloured subject.

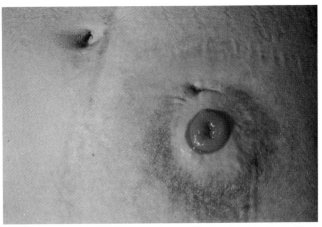

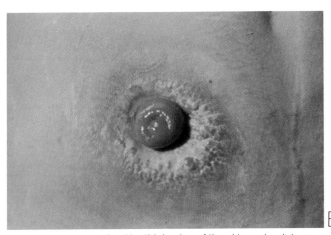

**Fig. 3.117 A, B.** Chronic phase of dermatitis due to chemical attack. This phase is characterized by thickening of the skin and a slate-grey colour (A) as well as by accentuation of the skin furrows and folds (B).

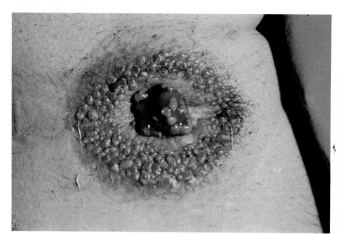

**Fig. 3.118.** Peristomal lichenization.

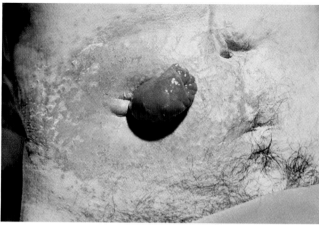

**Fig. 3.119.** Dermatitis all around a defective ileostomy. The stoma, in fact, points upwards and the faecal dicharge infiltrates beneath the appliance macerating the skin.

avoid situations which will make it unmanageable, i.e. situations such those in which liquid discharge and faeces are allowed to leak onto the surrounding skin and macerate it (Fig. 3.119).

Lastly, it is imperative to cleanse the peristomal skin with aqueous boric acid solutions, chloroxidants or, even better, by washing with water and acid soaps, i.e. the so-called «non-soaps».

# 4. Secondary stomal pathology

This chapter is devoted to a series of dieases of various kinds comprising in part stomal manifestations of generalized diseases such as portal hypertension and in part the localization or repetition on the stoma of intestinal diseases such as tumours or inflammatory and infectious diseases of the colon.

A special section is given over exclusively to the subject of pharmacological lesions, which are becoming increasingly frequent.

## PORTAL HYPERTENSION

A possible, albeit rare consequence of portal hypertension in ostomy patients is the formation of mucocutaneous varices in the stoma.

The phenomenon is more often present in the ileostomy, and in these cases the portal hypertension is due to cirrhosis secondary to the chronic inflammatory colopathy for which the stoma has been constructed,[14, 39] but mucocutaneous varices may also appear in a colostomy as a result of portal hypertension due to hepatic metastases of a rectal carcinoma.[30, 84]

Lastly, if we are in the presence of a cirrhosis which is independent of the disease which led to the construction of the intestinal diversion, the varices may appear regardless of the particular type of stoma.[43]

The small intestine and colon are not among the sites affected by formation of discharge shunts in cases of portal hypertension,[39] but, when a portion of bowel is exteriorized and joined up to the abdominal wall, a fresh possibility of anastomosis is created, by means of the epigastric veins, between the portal system and the vena cava inferior system with the formation of portosystemic shunts in the region of the mucocutaneous stoma junction.[2, 28]

The aspect of a varicose stoma is characteristic: the mucosa bulges with large venous vessels which run over into the surrounding skin, which is taut, thin, shiny and bluish in colour, and either spread out radially or pursue tortuous routes, creating an unmistakeable caput medusae with its centre in the stoma (Fig. 4.1). A rarer phenomenon is peristomal venular ectasia, which manifests itself as a purple circular area consisting of a dense network of small dilated vessels (Fig. 4.2).

From the clinical point of view, the main problem of stomal varices is haemorrhage. The varices, in fact, subjected as they are to continual traumatism as a result of cleansing manoeuvres and the constant changing of the stoma appliance, tend to erode easily, giving rise to bleeding which may be only of modest proportions, i.e. a slight, yet continuous stillicide, or, more often, to profuse haemorrhages which require transfusions and put the patient's life at risk.

The diagnosis is made by simple inspection, especially in patients in whom portal hypertension is already known and documented. It may, however, happen that the stomal varices constitute the first warning sign of portal hypertension and in such cases it is essential to ascertain the existence and proportions of the phenomenon, using a manometer, as well as the cause by means of a thorough study of the liver. The study of the splanchnic vascularization by both arteriography

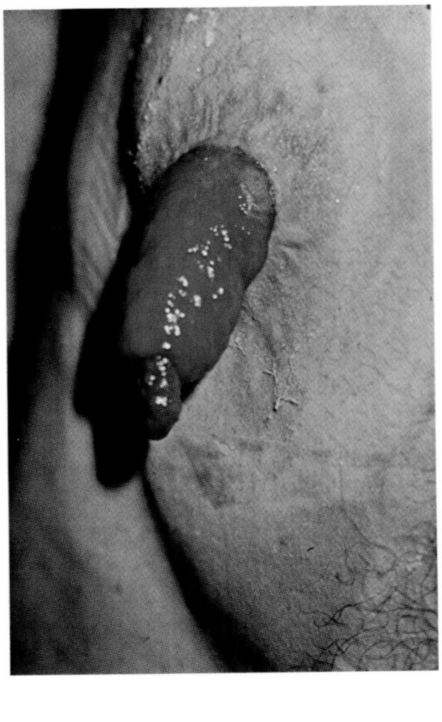

**Fig. 4.1.** Varices in an ileostomy performed for ulcerative colitis in a patient suffering from portal hypertension due to cirrhosis secondary to chronic inflammatory colopathy. The peristomal skin is shiny, thin and taut and the dilated venous vessels are detectable below the surface.

◀          ▶

**Fig. 4.2.** A rare photograph of peristomal venular dilatation at the base of an ileostomy constructed for polyposis of the colon. The phenomenon is secondary to portal hypertension induced by metastatic invasion of the liver.

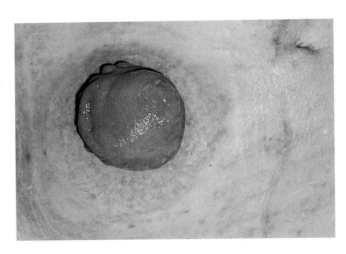

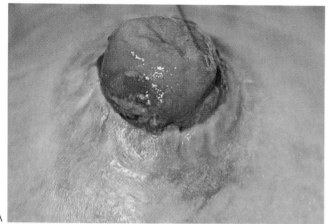

A

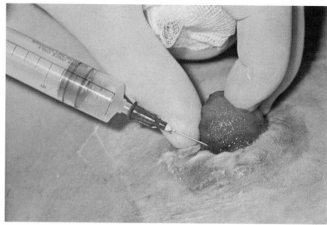

B

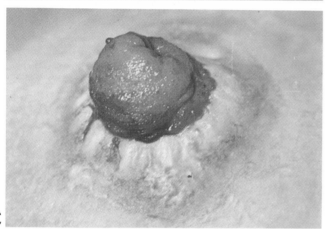

C

**Fig. 4.3 A, B, C.** A) Varices at the base of an ileostomy. The macroscopic aspect is that of caput medusae. A bleeding varix is visible on the mucocutaneous edge. B) Injection of sclerosing solution at the base of the stoma. C) Twenty-four hours after the injection of sclerosant solution, the haemorrhage has stopped. A marked peristomal inflammatory reaction may be noted.

and splenoportography serves the purpose of demonstrating definitely the causal relationship between the peristomal venous ectasias and the obstacle to portal flow.

The treatment of stomal varices is not simple, above all when the nature and degree of the liver disease responsible for the portal hypertension preclude radical surgery such as portosystemic diversions; the latter are the only measures capable of guaranteeing a regression of the varices, but are practicable only in cirrhotic patients.

Conversely, in patients with metastatic invasion of the liver, the only viable measures are symptomatic and of local character. They consist in haemostasis by compression or suture of the bleeding vessel.[30, 39, 94]

Another possibility is disconnection of the stoma accompanied by multiple peristomal ligatures and concluded with a new mucocutaneous suture.[14, 28]

The use of subcutaneous injections of sclerosant solutions[29] may be tried in the initial stages of the disease when the varices are not yet very extensive (Fig. 4.3 A, B, C). Finally, one may resort to the systemic infusion of vasopressin.[48]

It is, of course, always necessary to take steps to correct any coagulation disorders.

In any case, such measures provide only a temporary solution of the haemorrhage problem, which is inevitably bound to recur.

As far as the management of a varicose stoma is concerned, it goes without saying that the appliances used must be of the two-piece type equipped with soft flanges or washers so as to minimize the traumatisms.

It is imperative to avoid the use of stoma belts whose clips may injure the peristomal skin, and of additional support plasters.

In the haemorrhagic stage, appliances must be used with diameters large enough to accommodate the stoma and the skin area with the bleeding varices.

## NEOPLASIA

The neoplastic manifestations affecting the stoma include the original neoplasm, contemporaneous or subsequent neoplasm, recurrences, extrinsic compression and invasion due to contiguity.

These are infrequent situations prevalently affecting colostomies, though descriptions are to be found in literature of cases of neoplasm arising in an ileostomy or ureteroileocutaneostomy with thoroughly original hypotheses put forward with regard to their origin.[42, 59]

The appearance of the original neoplasm and of metachronous neoplasm is subordinate to the general causes of the cancerogenesis and thus cannot be prognosticated or prevented.

Conversely, the appearance of synchronous neoplasm and recurrence is almost always the result of a diagnostic or therapeutic error and thus could be avoided by a thorough study of the patient and extensive bowel resections at a safe distance from the original tumour.

Extrinsic compression and invasion of the stoma due to contiguity are due to the progressive evolution of the original lesion which has not been removed and manifest themselves in palliative colostomies some time after their construction.

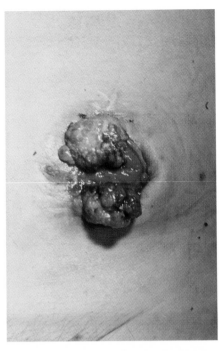

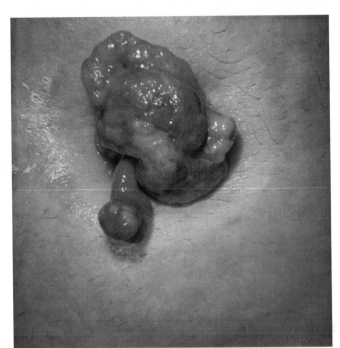

**Fig. 4.4.** Typical aspect of stomal neoplastic invasion. The neoplasm appears to be of multicentric origin. ◄

**Fig. 4.5.** Appearance of a large neoplastic polyp at the moment of opening a terminal sigmoidostomy after rectal excision for neoplasm. Once the ampullar lesion had been identified by digital exploration and rectoscopy, the examinations were suspended and the patient was immediately operated on. ►

◄

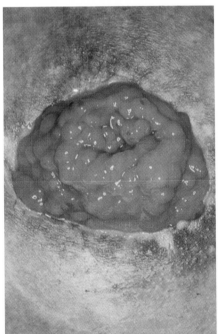

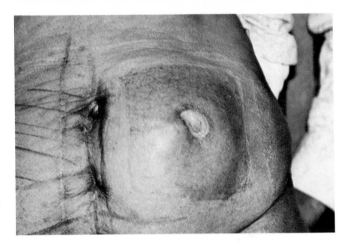

**Fig. 4.6.** Familial polyposis on a sigmoidostomy constructed five years earlier for carcinoma of the rectum. The patient had not come in for any further checks during the interim period. On this occasion the patient declined any form of therapy. ►

**Fig. 4.7.** Misalignment and extrinsic compression of a terminal sigmoid colostomy due to diffuse endo-abdominal neoplasm. (Infra-red ray photograph to show up the tumefactions).

The characteristic aspect of a stomal neoplasm is an efflorescence of neoplastic tissue gradually replacing the stomal mucosa (Fig. 4.4).

Synchronous tumours usually present in the form of single pedunculated polyps which manifest themselves immediately when the stoma is first constructed (Fig. 4.5) or may appear in a diffuse form covering the entire stoma (Fig. 4.6).

The stoma, moreover, may appear undamaged as regards the mucosa but proves to be misaligned or displaced owing to extrinsic compression caused by endoabdominal neoplastic masses (Fig. 4.7).

From the clinical point of view, stomal neoplasms may give rise to haemorrhages even of conspicuous proportions or render the stoma unserviceable owing to partial or complete obstruction of the orifice with consequent intestinal occlusion (Fig. 4.8).

The clinical picture, moreover, is completed by the appearance of a reaction of anguish typical of patients with external neoplasms when they can actually see their own disease.

The diagnosis in thus very easy and may be made by straightforward inspection. In the initial stages, however, a primitive or metachronous neoplasm or recurrence may be mistaken for a granuloma or any other type of productive inflammatory lesion. When dealing with any stomal neoformation, it is thus imperative to perform a biopsy.

From the therapeutic point of view, the chances of success are closely related to the type of neoplastic manifestation.

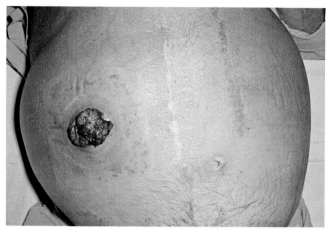

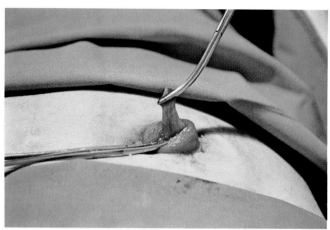

**Fig. 4.8.** Intestinal occlusion due to obstruction of a colostomy as a result of neoplastic invasion. In this case there is also coexistent ascites.

**Fig. 4.9.** Resection of a polyp protruding from a terminal sigmoidostomy.

In primary and metachronous neoplasms and in recurrences radical surgical treatment is possible, consisting in extensive resections together with the construction of a new stoma on a proximal segment.

When, as often happens in the case of synchronous neoplasms, the lesion takes the form of a polyp, the latter is excised and a thorough endoscopic and radiological study is made of the residual colon (Fig. 4.9). In the absence of other polyps, one need do no more than ensure constant, thorough surveillance of the patient's condition.

Conversely, in the case of extrinsic compression or invasion of the stoma due to contiguity, the therapeutic possibilities are limited. These, in fact, are patients in the terminal stage with diffuse carcinoma, in whom nothing more can be done than put a stop to any haemorrhages by electrocoagulation or temporarily restore canalization by means of partial excision of neoplastic tissue or the construction of a second stoma higher up. It should not, however, be forgotten that this latter measure often proves ineffective because the proximal intestinal segments are frequently subject to the endoperitoneal diffusion of the neoplasm.

## INFLAMMATORY COLOPATHIES

Enterostomies, and particularly the ileostomy, constitute what is virtually the inevitable conclusion of inflammatory colopathy care and, therefore, the only relationship between enterostomies and inflammatory colopathies must necessarily be a purely casual one. Conversely, there are certain conditions in which the stoma is affected by lesions peculiar to both ulcerative colitis and Crohn's disease.

*Ileostomy.* In ulcerative colitis an ileostomy may be subject to so-called postcolectomy ileitis,[91] which is either localized in the stomal mucosa alone or extends to one or more loops of the adjoining small intestine.

Among the stomal forms, apart from ischaemia-based forms or those due to stenosis, the most common is reflux ileitis[62] due to the fact that prior to the colostomy there was repeated contact between the ileal mucosa and the contents of the diseased colon which re-ascended to the last loop owing to insufficiency of the ileocecal valve. It is, therefore, the expression of a conceptual error consisting in the use of a portion of diseased bowel to construct the stoma.

The stoma appears hyperaemic, oedematous and even ulcerated, sometimes covered with fibrin patches (Fig. 4.10).

This form of ileitis usually heals spontaneously and all that is necessary is to fit the stoma with very soft appliances or even leave it without an appliance.

If the mucosal lesions do not regress within a few days, the stoma must be refashioned, using a healthy portion of bowel.

Prestomal ileitis, on the other hand, be it acute or latent,[91] is a serious disease of a perforative chatacter, which is well known from both the clinical and morphological points of view but is still obscure from the aetiological point of view (Fig. 4.11). During the period preceding the actual outbreak of the disease, the stoma may be affected by pathological phenomena such as retraction or the formation of fistulas, which are usually put down to technical errors and may even be corrected as such, whereas, in fact, they are bound up with the ileitis, which has not as yet clearly manifested itself.

In the acute stage, the stomal repercussions consist in congestion of the mucosa and an increase in the quantity of discharge, which is unmistakeably watery and foul-smelling (Fig. 4.12). This form may only be treated surgically by eliminating the diseased portion of bowel.

In Crohn's disease the ileostomy may be affected by relapses or by peristomal skin lesions consisting in fistulas and so-called metastatic forms.[70]

The relapses present no particular characteristics apart from the fact that they are often mistaken for cases of postcolectomy ileitis.

The most common skin lesions which manifest

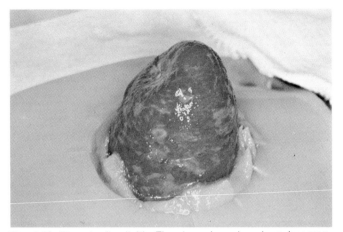

**Fig. 4.10.** Stomal reflux ileitis. The stoma is oedematous, hyperaemic, ulcerated and covered with pseudo-membranes. The stoma is fitted with a very soft flange and the base is surrounded with protective paste.

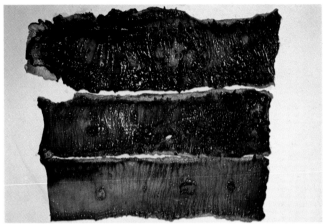

**Fig. 4.11.** Prestomal ileitis. Multiple ileal resections for a very severe form of a necrotizing, haemorrhagic nature, arising three years after a colectomy.

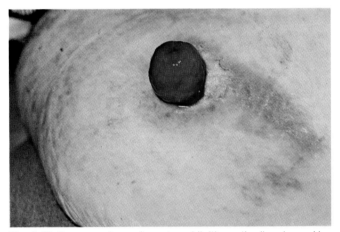

**Fig. 4.12.** Repercussions of prestomal ileitis on the ileostomy. Hyperaemia and congestion of the mucosa. The peristomal ecchymosis is due to a rigid ileostomy appliance which the patient managed to keep stuck to the skin by applying excessive pressure in an attempt to stem the enormous quantity of watery discharge.

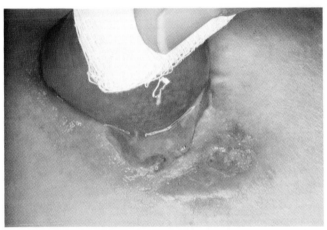

**Fig. 4.13.** Viscerocutaneous fistula at the base of an ileostomy in a patient subjected to colectomy for Crohn's disease.

themselves in cases of relapse of Crohn's disease are fistulas. They are the typical viscerocutaneous fistulas of Crohn's disease and emerge in the vicinity of the stoma (Fig. 4.13), and their continual secretions make normal stoma management impossible.

In this case, too, local treatment is no use and the fistulas will only heal after resection has been performed.

The so-called metastatic skin forms, which are rather rare, break down into two distinct groups.[71] The first comprises a whole series of dermatoses of varying aetiology, the most prominent of which are pyoderma gangrenosum, erythema nodosum and acne erythematosa.

The second group is made up of erosive lesions (Fig. 4.14) which present a sarcoid reaction[70] with epithelioid and Langhans-type cells grouped together in non-caseous granulomas inserted in chronic inflammatory tissue.[71]

These peristomal lesions may accompany an ileal relapse of the disease,[87] constitute a serious problem with regard to stoma management and fail to benefit from local treatment.

*Colostomy.* No type of colostomy should ever be the site of an inflammatory colopathy providing the latter does not occur suddenly in a patient given a colostomy for other reasons.

In the surgical treatment of ulcerative and granulomatous colitis, in fact, it is always preferable to avoid a colostomy on which the disease might easily continue to manifest itself or reappear after a period of latency.

It may happen, however, that a simple diverting colostomy is resorted to in order to cure untreatable anal fistulas mistakenly judged to be aspecific or colectasia overhastily attributed to obstruction.

In such cases, the lesions characteristic of the unrecognized colopathy will promptly appear on the stoma.

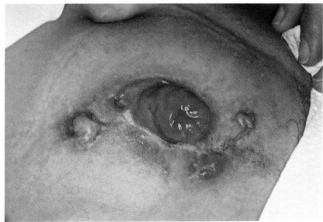

**Fig. 4.14.** So-called metastatic skin lesions in a patient given an ileostomy for Crohn's disease. There is also coexistent distress of the mucosa, which appears to be bleeding.

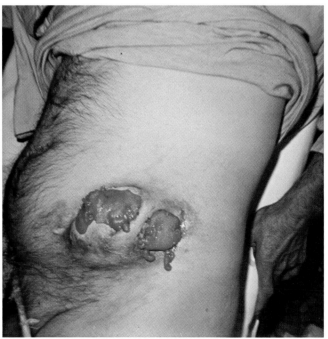

**Fig. 4.15.** Productive lesions typical of Crohn's disease on a diverting skin-bridge colostomy constructed for anal fistulas which were locally untreatable and judged to be aspecific.

In Crohn's disease they manifest a typical productive character with exuberance of the mucosa and the formation of granulomas (Fig. 4.15).

In ulcerative colitis, the aspect is that of a colostomy covered with hyperaemic, bleeding mucosa. Losses of substance appear at the mucocutaneous margin and their development parallels the progressive decline in general condition leading eventually to atrophy of the

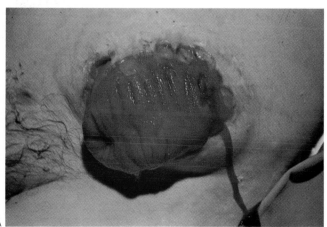

A

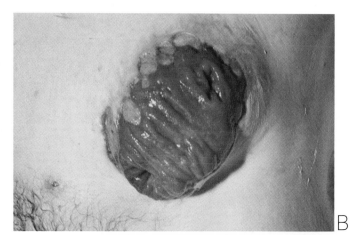

B

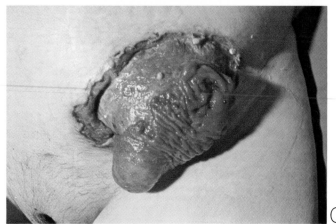

C

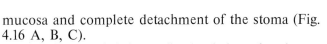

**Fig. 4.16 A, B, C.** A) Sigmoid colostomy constructed for a dilatation of the colon judged to be of an obstructive nature. Actually, the patient was suffering from ulcerative colitis. The mucosa is oedematous and congested and bleeds profusely. B) A few days later the mucosa tends towards atrophy. Evident loss of substance may be noted around the mucocutaneous edge. C) Terminal phase: complete atrophy of the mucosa and spontaneous visceroparietal detachment due to dysprotidaemia and debility of the patient.

mucosa and complete detachment of the stoma (Fig. 4.16 A, B, C).

In both cases, it is immediately obvious that the colostomy has proved to be of no use as regards improving the clinical pattern, which continues to take its

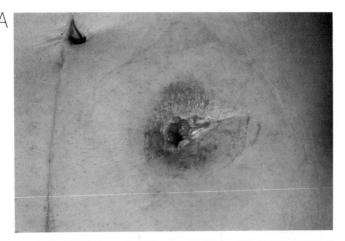

A

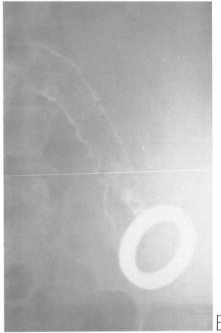

B

**Fig. 4.17 A, B, C, D.**
A) Magnetic left terminal colostomy constructed at the end of a Miles operation for presumed rectal neoplasm. Actually, the condition was ampullar localization of Crohn's disease. A few months after surgery the stoma presented retracted, suppurating and surrounded by an intense skin reaction. B) A barium enema revealed the existence and extent of the colopathy. C) Operative portion of residual colectomy with removal of the magnetic ring. D) Postoperative aspect. There is now a definitive ileostomy.

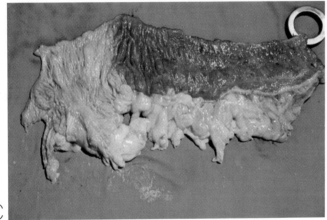

C

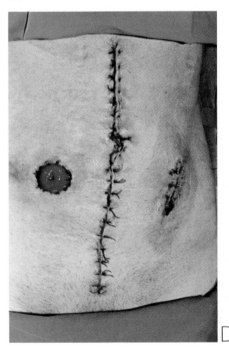

D

natural course and, what is more, is complicated by the disorders induced by a diseased stoma.

Actually seeing the disease on the stomal mucosa should hasten the use of the only therapeutic resource available, consisting in the removal of the colon, and thus of the colostomy, and the construction of an ileostomy (Fig. 4.17 A, B, C, D).

## INFECTIOUS AND PARASITIC DISEASES

Infectious and parasitic diseases are only exceptionally responsible for stomal alterations. When the latter occur, they are wholly aspecific and consist in hyperaemia and congestion of the stoma, which tends to bleed easily.

An exception to this rule is amoebiasis, which, by contrast, gives rise to specific lesions characterized by tissue destruction.

The stoma may be involved as a result of contiguity or may be directly affected.

In the former case, the histolysis of the abdominal wall brought about by the parasite may spread to a point where it borders on the stoma, which remains intact but cannot easily have an appliance fitted on account of the lack of sufficient skin surface to take the stoma appliance flange (Fig. 4.18).

If, on the other hand, the stoma is directly involved, it bleeds profusely, retracts and tends to detach itself from the skin eroded by the amoebas and in the throes of severe irritation of a vesicular type (Fig. 4.19 A, B, C, D).

Another eventuality, albeit somewhat rare, consists in the appearance of an amoebic granuloma on the stoma (Fig. 4.20).

These situations are typical of cases in which the bowel resection is performed on the basis of a generic diagnosis of acute perforative colopathy or toxic colectasia without the surgeon's being aware of the presence

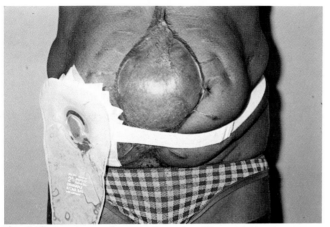

**Fig. 4.18.** Ileostomy after colectomy for diffuse fulminating amoebic colitis. After the operation, a vast area of abdominal wall has been eroded by the amoebas. The residual defect is covered only by the skin.

of amoeba; the resection is thus not immediately followed by specific pharmacological therapy, which, once introduced, is capable of bringing about complete regression both of the skin and stomal lesions.

## PHARMACOLOGICAL LESIONS

The adverse effects of many categories of drugs on the alimentary tract mucosa or on the consolidation processes of surgical wounds are by now well known.

Enterostomies, by their very nature, are particularly subject to such effects and, in actual fact, the cases of

**Fig. 4.19 A, B, C, D.** A left terminal colostomy in the throes of amoebic infection (A). The lesions had appeared shortly after construction of the ileostomy for perforation of the sigmoid (B), the nature of which was detected only by histological examination (C). After initiating specific medical therapy, the lesions regress in a few days (D).

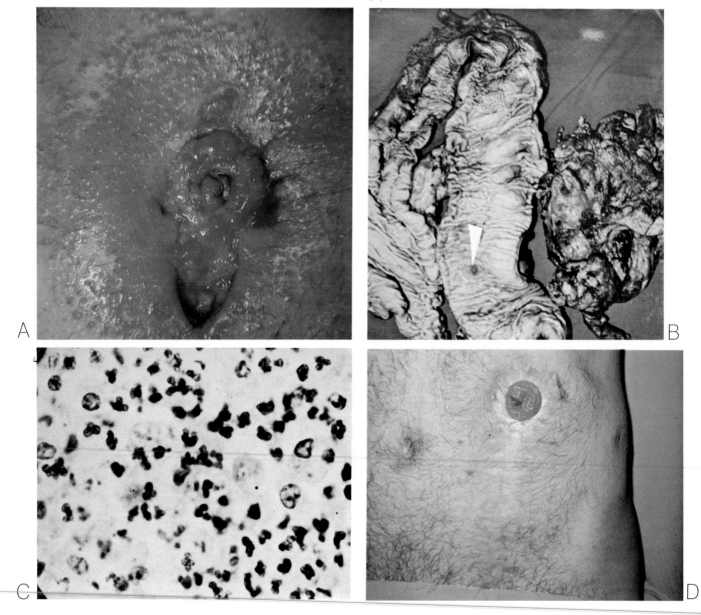

severe stomal alterations secondary to the administration of various drugs are by no means rare.

Among those drugs capable of giving rise to appreciable lesions, the most prominent are analgesic-anti-inflammatory drugs, corticosteroids, immunosuppressants, cytotoxics and antibiotics.

The most frequent pathological manifestations in

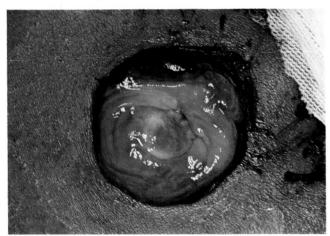

**Fig. 4.20.** Amoebic granuloma in the 7 o'clock position on an ileostomy in the throes of ischaemic distress.

this connection are mucosal haemorrhages and visceroparietal detachment.

Mucosal haemorrhages constitute the characteristic effect of prolonged therapy based on the use of analgesic-anti-inflammatory drugs. Such haemorrhages may also be of considerable proportions and are due primarily to the inhibition of platelet aggregation induced by salicylates, indomethacin and other drugs belonging to this category.

The stoma becomes congested and transudation occurs without any disruption of the mucosa being detectable (Fig. 4.21).

The diagnosis is based on inspection and on the

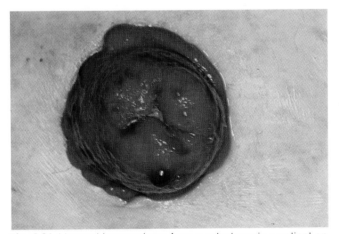

**Fig. 4.21.** Mucosal haemorrhage from a colostomy in a patient on long-term indomethacin treatment. The blood is oozing out of a mucosa which is macroscopically intact, but congested and hyperaemic.

anamnestic datum relating to the taking of analgesic-anti-inflammatory drugs in the past. The diagnosis must be completed by a coagulation study and, particularly, by a study of platelet aggregation capability. Obviously, one should first exclude the presence of other sources of mucosal haemorrhage throughout the alimentary tract, especially at the gastric level.

In the bleeding phase, stoma appliances should not be fitted and the stoma should be covered with gauze or cotton wool soaked in coagulant solutions or simply in cold water.

Should the use of a stoma appliance prove absolutely indispensable, the appliance must be very soft and must be fitted with great care and delicacy.

As far as the evolution of these haemorrhages is concerned, cessation of the drug and readjustment of the coagulation process usually put a stop to the haemorrhage quite rapidly.

Stomal haemorrhages may also occur during cycles of therapy with cytotoxics. In this case, the phenomenon is related to the thrombocytopenia which accompanies the leukopenia and anaemia induced by this category of drugs. The stomal mucosa thus appears pale rather than congested and hyperaemic, but bleeds all the same (Fig. 4.22 A, B). In this case, too, administration of the drug must be temporarily suspended and the equilibrium of the patient's blood supply re-established by transfusion.

The visceroparietal detachment, or rather the failure of the exteriorized loop to adhere to the abdominal wall, is, on the other hand, a possible effect of the administration of corticosteroids and immunosoppressants which interfere with the so-called inflammatory phase in the healing of wounds. It is an extremely dangerous occurrence and is difficult to remedy as it usually occurs in patients in whom the steroid and immunosuppressant therapy cannot be interrupted. The result is that the detachment of the stoma progresses rapidly, especially if there is a coexistent structural defect, to the point of complete disjunction, occasionally with associated dehiscence of the main incision (Fig. 4.23 A, B, C).

The administration of cytotoxic drugs may also cause peristomal erosions which may go so far as to bring about actual detachment (Fig. 4.24 A, B).

The stomal lesions induced by cytotoxics are, however, more sluggish in their development than those caused by corticosteroids or immunosuppressants; they progress more slowly and, in addition, respond positively to the cyclic suspension of the drug, thereby tending to undergo periodic regression.

The possibility therefore exists of treating the loss of peristomal substance by filling in the eroded areas with soft, plastic, inert materials. The stoma is then fitted with karaya washers, to which large-sized drainable bags can be made to adhere perfectly, thereby preventing the faecal discharge from collecting in the peristomal recess and contaminating it (Fig. 4.25 A, B, C).

As the lost substance is gradually made up, on restoring the cell stock in the blood by suspending the

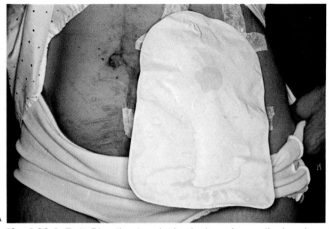
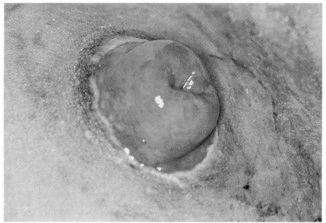

**Fig. 4.22 A, B.** A) Bleeding terminal colostomy in a patient undergoing therapy with cytotoxic drugs. B) With the appliance removed, the stoma is pale in appearance due to anaemia induced by the drug. The aspect is quite different from that in Fig. 4.21.

chemotherapy, the residual cavity may be packed with bismuth iodoform gauze, which stimulates the granulation processes (Fig. 4.26 A, B, C).

Instead of iodoform gauze one can use karaya paste, which sets on contact with the air and may be overlaid with a protective barrier, thus making for perfect stoma management (Fig. 4.27 A, B).

Healing will be achieved only by virtue of repeated, patient medication and on condition that the administration of cytostatic drugs is suspended (Fig. 4.28 A, B).

A special situation obtains in relation to the use of antibiotics.

The indiscriminate use of antibiotics both in hospital wards and elsewhere must needs be considered responsible for the conspicuous increase in forms of bacterial enterocolitis registered over the past few years. A very serious example of this is, without doubt, pseudomembranous colitis associated with the use of various antibiotics, particularly clindamycin and lincomycin.[6, 25]

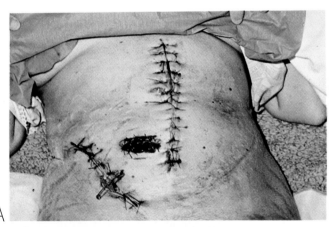
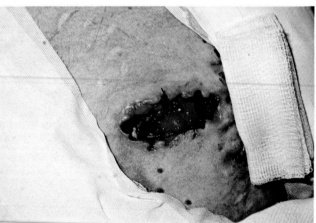

**Fig. 4.23 A, B, C.** A) Mikulicz colostomy for spontaneous perforation of the colon in a young woman subjected to double kidney transplant with rejection of the right transplanted kidney. The patient was receiving high doses of cortisone and immunosuppressives, the steroids being the probable cause of the perforated colon. B) 48 hours after its construction, the colostomy presented retracted and detached, amongst other things owing to substantial tension on the exteriorized loop. C) Complete detachment of the colostomy and dehiscence of the main wound at day 7.

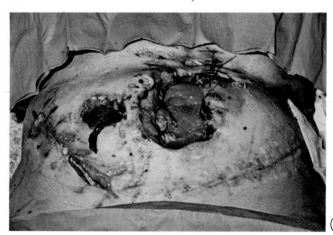

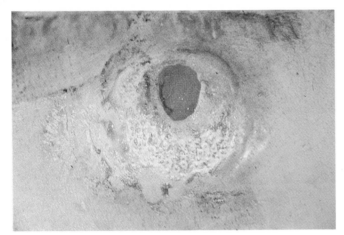

**Fig. 5.11.** Peristomal radiodermatitis.

prudent distribution of the rays, makes it possible to avoid dermatitis even in patients with sensitive skin (Fig. 5.13 A, B).

A final set of problems are those relating to particularly troublesome intestinal dysfunctions in patients lacking voluntary control of evacuation.

In subjects who make abundant use of analgesics, an obstinate form of constipation usually sets in requiring periodic intestinal irrigation in order to remove faecalomas, which can actually cause occlusion if trapped in a rigid, stenotic bowel segment. Further to this, oral stool softeners and propellants may be prescribed.

In other patients, the occurrence of diarrhoea and enteritis with malabsorption is more frequent. The use of intestinal astringents is indicated only if the radiology has not revealed radiation-induced organic alterations. In this case the solution is surgical and consists in resection or by-pass of the small intestine.

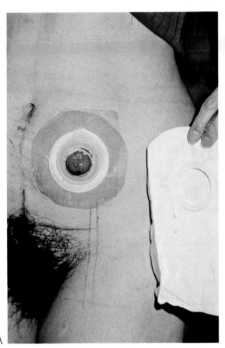

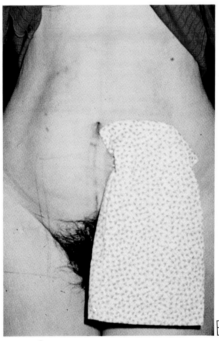

A      B

**Fig. 5.12 A, B.** A) A two-piece appliance fitted on a patient due to undergo radiation. B) To avoid contact between the sensitized skin and the plastic of the bag, a cotton cover is used.

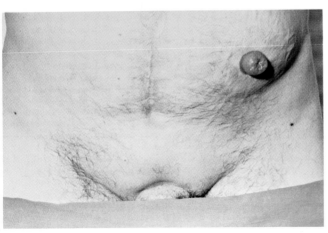

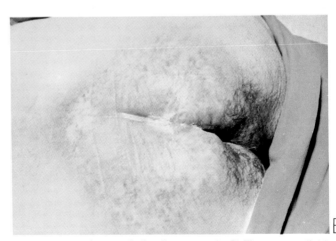

A      B

**Fig. 5.13 A, B.** A) Taking all due precautions, the peristomal skin proves undamaged after a radiation therapy cycle. B) The same patient was subjected, one year later, to a further cycle of radiotherapy of the perineal region for a recurrence. On that occasion, the radiation brought about severe dermatitis due to failure to apply the standard care and prevention procedures.

# 6. Stomal problems in gynaecology and obstetrics

In addition to problems of a general nature and those connected with radiotherapy to which female ostomy patients are often subjected for gynaecological diseases, they must also face particular problems resulting from the site of the original disease. Prominent among these are problems of a sexual character ranging from the temporary suspension of sexual activity, as in the case of rectovaginal fistulas, to the permanent inability to have sexual relations, as in the case of tumours of the vulva (Fig. 6.1 A, B).

From the psychological point of view such situations have negative repercussions which end up by sapping the patient's will to recover with the result that these patients require special psychological assistance.

Also of a very particular nature are the problems an ostomy patient is liable to encounter in the obstetric field, that is to say when she decides to undertake a pregnancy.

For obvious reasons relating to age and the prognosis of the original disease, practically speaking, the problem concerns only patients with an ileostomy for inflammatory colopathy, but at the same time we cannot rule out cases involving patients with colostomies or urostomies for neoplasms.

Pregnancy in ileostomy patients is a rare occurrence. The cases reported in literature over the past twenty years amount to just over a hundred,[20] although from the few published studies on the subject it may be deduced that the objective impediments to conception are very rare and the risks involved in gestation and child-birth controllable.

The explanation of the rarity of the phenomenon, therefore, lies in fears resulting from an approximate knowledge of the problem, leading ileostomy patients to give up the idea and doctors to dissuade such patients from undertaking a pregnancy.

The only actual contraindication may be kidney insufficiency due to the lithiasis which not infrequently accompanies ileostomy.

In patients operated on for Crohn's disease we should add the dangers of relapses or persistance of the disease in the residual ampulla of the rectum or in the perineum.

For this reason pregnancy must not be undertaken unless healing is guaranteed and thus not before a year has elapsed since the operation.

Conception may be impeded by factors which depend on the original disease, by the effects of the medical therapy applied prior to the operation or by the outcome of the operation itself.

Forms of adnexitis secondary to the propagation of the colonic inflammation to the organs of the lesser pelvis and the side effects of prolonged cortisone therapy may protract the reduction in fertility already demonstrated in the acute phase of the disease.[63]

Surgery may give rise to adhesion processes which

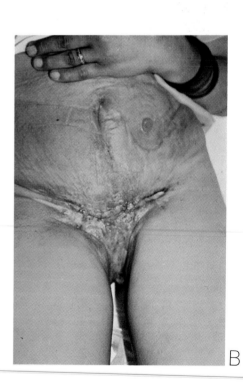

**Fig. 6.1 A, B.** A) Neoplasm of the vulva extending to the anus. B) Following excision and radiation, the patient was unable to have sexual relations, thereby adding further limitations to those already associated with the stoma.

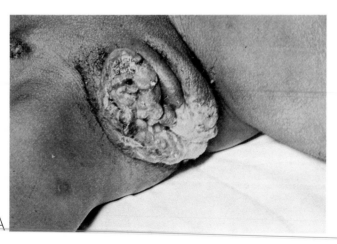

A

B

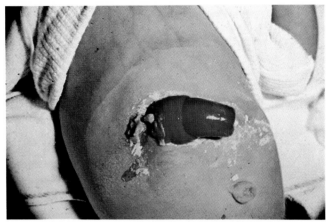

Fig. 7.6. Intussusception of the prolapsed distal loop of a double-barrelled colostomy. The proximal loop is functionally viable.

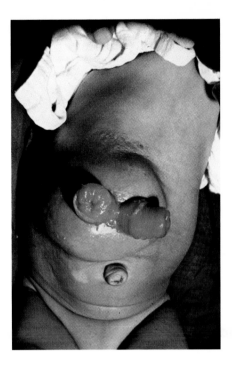

Fig. 7.7. Peristomal hernia and transverse colosromy prolapse. ▶

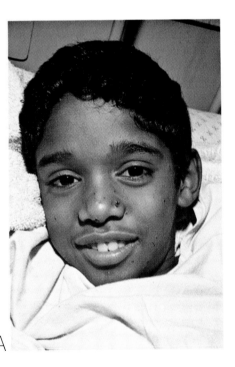

Fig. 7.8 A, B. A) Child operated on for an anal malformation and suffering from chicken-pox. B) The varicella lesions are also evident on the prolapsed stomal mucosa.

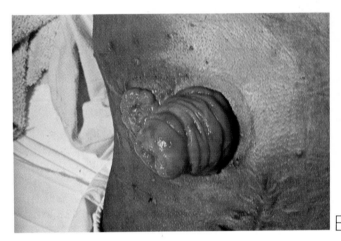

A

B

from secondary diseases; we may, for example, observe the presence of exanthema on the stoma in the course of infectious diseases (Fig. 7.8 A, B).

## Urostomies

The widespread use of intermittent catheterization, particularly in male infants with a neurogenic bladder due to spina bifida, has substantially reduced the frequency of urostomies in infancy. There are, however, enough to justify some mention of their main problems.

The first problem concerns the stoma site, which must be chosen, bearing in mind the fact that urostomies are generally permanent fixtures.

The disturbances resulting from their unmanageaability are therefore bound to be long-lasting and may prove so troublesome as to require extremely demanding surgical correction (Fig. 7.9 A, B).

Also of particular importance is the problem of urinary dermatitis, for the healing of which we must use boric or zinc-based powders so as to restore the cutaneous pH.

As in the case of enterostomies, these forms of dermatitis are exacerbated by poor siting of the stoma (Fig. 7.10).

In addition, the infant urostomy patient may be prone to a whole series of general, septic and metabolic complications, the diagnosis of which requires constant urinary, haematological and radiological checks.

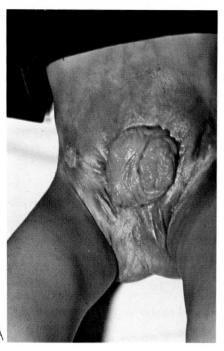

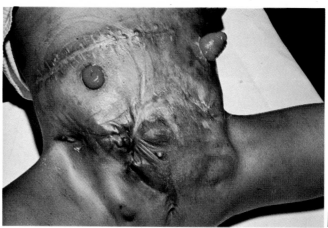

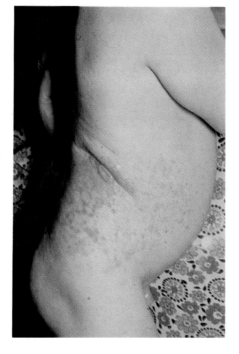

A

B

**Fig. 7.9 A, B.** A) Prolapsed caecostomy and poorly sited flush urostomy close to the iliac crest, constructed for ageneses of the perineal orifices. The urostomy is unmanageable. B) After surgical correction, a well-constructed ileostomy is visible on the left replacing the caecostomy together with an easily manageable ileal loop diversion on the right.

As regards the urostomy appliance, only those of the tap drainable type should be used; in livelier infants, the use of a urostomy belt is advisable. A correct choice of appliance will solve the problem of disagreeable odours and will save the child the embarrassment of being derided by other children of the same age.

Lastly, there is the problem of psychological damage. This problem can be solved only by tackling it on three fronts: 1) the child himself must be encouraged to become fully independent as soon as possible; 2) the parents must receive appropriate instruction as to the tasks involved in discreet supervision of the child; 3) teachers must be informed of the child's condition and needs, so that he will not be hindered at school if he needs to drink or go to the toilet.

**Fig. 7.10.** Urinary dermatitis around a lumbar sited – and therefore barely manageable – double ureterocutaneostomy. One of the two orifices is visibly larger than the other (megaureter).

# 8. Pathology in continent stomata

Ever since 1871, the year in which Schoenborn first suggested inserting a plug into a stoma, attempts at achieving voluntary control of evacuation in ostomy patients have multiplied.

The proposals put forward include methods based on external prosthetic appliances, intestinal plastic surgery and methods involving the implantation of active and passive prostheses.[89]

In actual fact, none of these has achieved the objective with the result that the continence sector continues to prove extremely stimulating.

Nevertheless, among the methods proposed over the past few years, there are two, namely the Kock intra-abdominal reservoir with nipple valve and the MACLET magnetic colostomy system, which have yielded such satisfactory results and have been adopted to such an extent that currently they may be considered synonymous with continence in the ileostomy and colostomy respectively.

Since they were first introduced, these methods have been modified and perfected; much has been written about them and the indications and operating techniques have been codified. Despite failures en route, the results now seem to have plateaued at acceptable levels, though at the same time it has equally become clear that there is a whole range of pathological conditions and diseases which are intimately bound up with their structure and functioning.

These are situations of varying degrees of seriousness, which may do no more than annul the effects of the device purporting to guarantee continence or may even go so far as to compromise the patient's health.

## ILEOSTOMY WITH INTRA-ABDOMINAL RESERVOIR AND NIPPLE-VALVE

The pathological situations which may affect this type of ileostomy are very closely related to the complexity of the operation.[40]

They include mechanical, inflammatory, ischaemic and traumatic manifestations, amounting to a fairly high total in all and with a mortality rate of approximately 2%.[37]

*Valvular dysfunctions*, which are, strictly speaking, mechanical accidents, constitute, the most frequent pathological situation and consist in the partial or complete extrusion of the nipple valve or its displacement.

In the case of extrusion, the valve gives way either partially (Fig. 8.1 A, B) or completely (Fig. 8.2); in the case of valve displacement, the valve, though remaining intact, is extroverted out of the reservoir and can be put back into the reservoir with appropriate manoeuvres.[84]

The cause lies in the yielding of the valve fixation sutures on the mesenteric side, which is always the

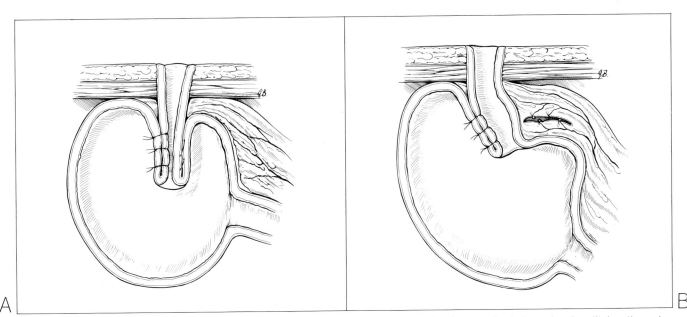

**Fig. 8.1 A, B.** A) Sectional diagram of a reservoir. B) Partial extrusion of the valve despite the expedient of passing the stitches through a mesenteric opening.

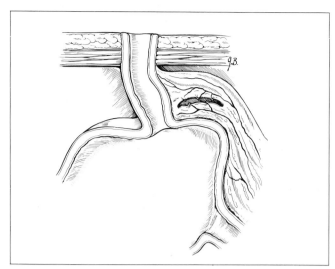

**Fig. 8.2.** Total extrusion.

In the case of partial extrusion, double-contrast radiology shows only a short, asymmetrical hint of a valve (Fig. 8.3 A, B) inside the reservoir.

In complete extrusion, the valve has disappeared altogether and, once the catheter used for the insufflation of contrast medium and air has been withdrawn, a long, tortuous conduit is observed corresponding to the evaginated portion of ileum leading from the abdominal wall to the reservoir (Fig. 8.4 A, B).

In the case of displacement, the valve appears normal when the catheter is in place but disappears as soon as it is withdrawn (Fig. 8.5 A, B).

Endoscopy, too, is of assistance in diagnosing valvular dysfunctions; the endoscopic pictures of partial extrusion, complete extrusion and displacement are just as characteristic as the radiological pictures and consist respectively in a short valve stump (Fig. 8.6 A, B), complete absence of the valve (Fig. 8.7 A, B) and mobility

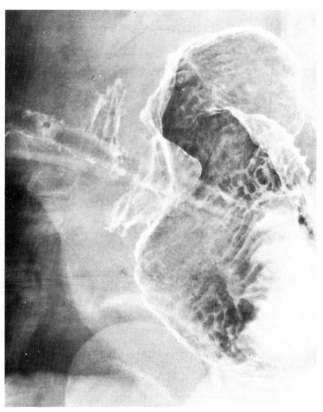

A

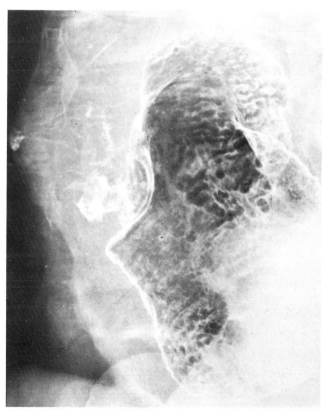

B

**Fig. 8.3 A, B.** Radiological pictures of partial extrusion of the valve. On introducing the catheter into the reservoir (A), a hint of a valve can be seen which disappears when the catheter is withdrawn (B). (By courtesy of Professor C.G. Standertskjöld-Nordenstam of the Department of Radiology of Helsinki University; from Br. J. Surg. 66: 269, 1979).

weakest point in the system despite the special techniques adopted to counteract it.[61]

The clinical pattern is characteristic: at a distance of a few weeks or months from the operation, the ileostomy patient begins to encounter difficulty in introducing the catheter. Soon afterwards, slight leakages of gas and mucus occur and ultimately spontaneous outflow of liquid discharge occurs.

of the valve in and out of the reservoir (Fig. 8.8 A, B).

All these situations require immediate surgical correction.

In complete extrusion, this may be confined to the reconstruction of the valve after first re-opening the reservoir (Fig. 8.9 A, B, C - Fig. 8.10 A, B), but in the other cases we must resort to surgical operations of substantial difficulty if we wish to avoid demolishing the

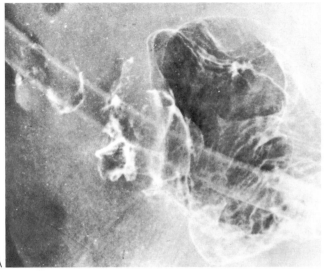

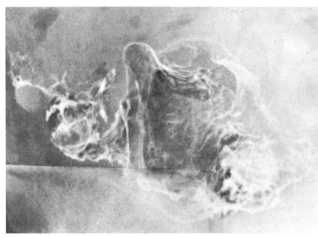

A                                                                                                          B

**Fig. 8.4 A, B.** Radiological pictures of total extrusion of the valve. The valve is not visible either on introducing the catheter into the reservoir (A) or on withdrawing it (B). (By courtesy of Professor C.G. Standertskjöld-Nordenstam of the Department of Radiology of Helsinki University: from Br. J. Surg. 66: 269, 1979).

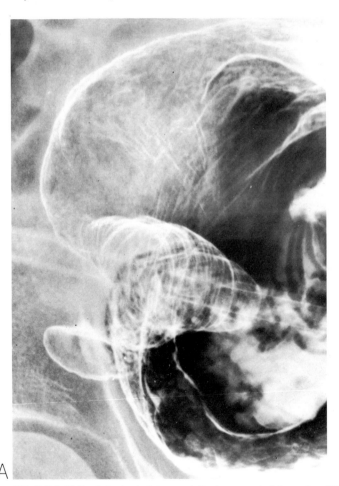

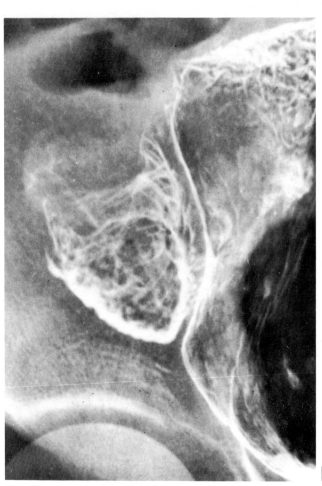

A                                                                                                          B

**Fig. 8.5 A, B.** Radiological pictures of displacement of the valve. When the catheter is introduced into the reservoir (A) the valve appears normal, whereas it disappears when the catheter is withdrawn (B). (By courtesy of Professor C.G. Standertskjöld-Nordenstam of the Department of Radiology of Helsinky University: from Br. J. Surg. 66: 269, 1979).

reservoir, thereby sacrificing a precious portion of bowel. These operations consist in resection of the valve, rotation of the reservoir and construction of a new continence mechanism[61] (Fig. 8.11 A, B, C, D) or, alternatively, in the replacement of the defective valve with another created by interposing an isolated ileal loop immediately upstream from the reservoir, which in this case is not rotated (Fig. 8.12 A, B, C).

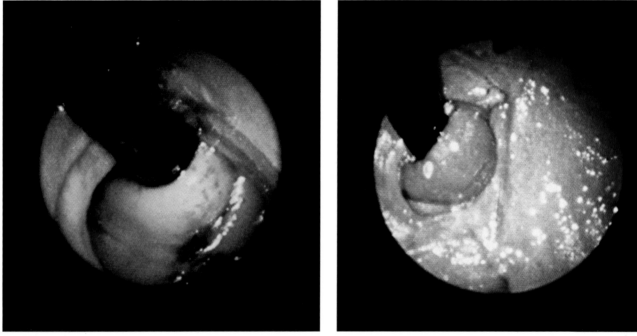

A                            B

**Fig. 8.6.** Retroversion endoscopy pictures of partial extrusion of the valve. Only a short portion of valve is sketchily outlined within the reservoir. (By courtesy of Professor J.D. Waye of the Mount Sinai Hospital, New York).

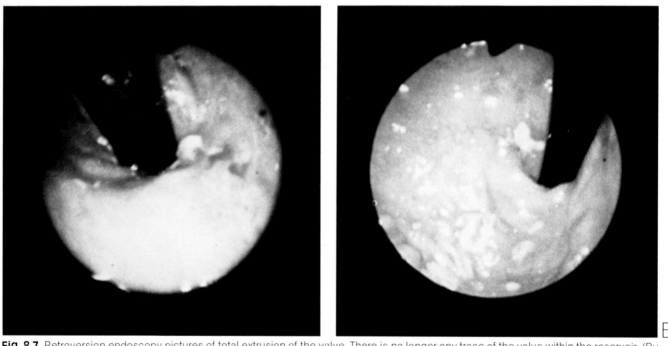

A                            B

**Fig. 8.7.** Retroversion endoscopy pictures of total extrusion of the valve. There is no longer any trace of the valve within the reservoir. (By courtesy of Professor J.D. Waye of the Mount Sinai Hospital, New York).

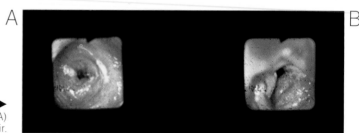

A                            B

**Fig. 8.8 A, B.** Endoscopic pictures of the mouth of the valve: in A) the valve is completely extroverted, in B) it is back in the reservoir.

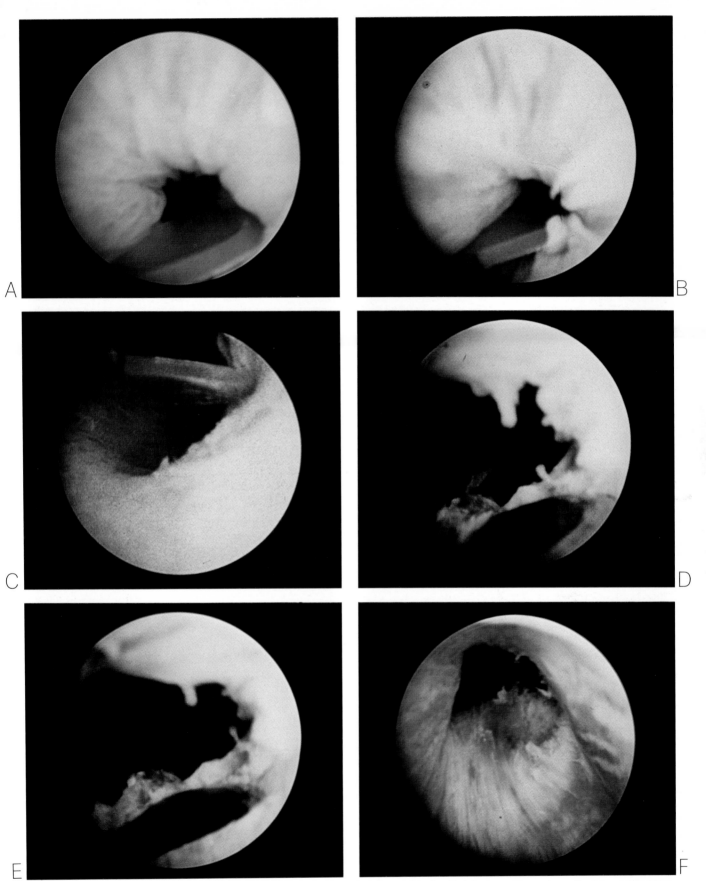

**Fig. 9.3 A, B, C, D, E, F.** Sequence of an endoscopic incision of the bladder neck in the 5 o'clock position using a Sachse urethrotome.

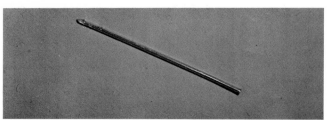

**Fig. 9.4.** Catheter for intermittent self-catheterization.

and organic impotence may, in turn, be either of a neurological or vascular nature.

To recognize the various forms we must perform a series of tests which constitute the current basis for the diagnosis of impairment of male sexual function.

N.P.T.M. (Nocturnal Penile Tumescence Monitoring) is used in order to distinguish between psychogenic and organic impotence. Patients suffering from the

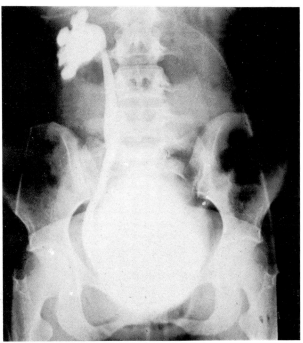
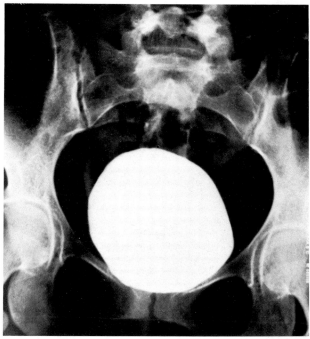

**Fig. 9.5 A, B.** Cytographic check on a patient subjected to amputation of the rectum: A) initial situation; B) after six months of intermittent self-catherization, the vesico-urethral reflux has almost completely disappeared and there is a marked improvement in the vesical morphology.

alpha-sympathicomimetic drugs (phenylpropanolamine, ephedrine) prior to sexual intercourse.

As already mentioned, the second type of dysfunction, i.e. impotence, may be psychogenic or organic,

former, in fact, are unable to suppress their nocturnal erections and therefore register a normal trace on the monitor, whereas those suffering from organic impotence present an absolutely flat trace (Fig. 9.6).

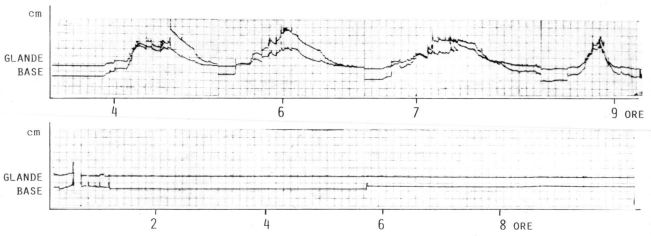

**Fig. 9.6.** N.P.T.M. (Nocturnal Penile Tumescence Monitoring). The top trace is that of a normal patient; the bottom trace is that of a patient suffering from organic impotence.

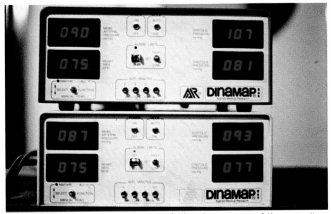

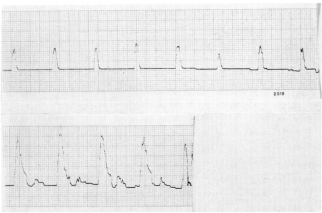

**Fig. 9.7.** Continuous monitoring of blood pressure of the arm (top monitor) and penis (bottom monitor). Each monitor records four values, namely:
Mean B.P. - Systolic B.P. - Heart Rate - Diastolic B.P.
In normal subjects the ratio of brachial to penile blood pressure is, practically speaking, 1:1, whereas in impotent patients it is greater than 1:1.

**Fig. 9.8.** Doppler flowmetry of the dorsal artery of the penis (top) as compared to that of the brachial artery (bottom) in a normal subject. The systolic blood pressure value is 130 mm in both regions. The brachio-penile pressure index is equal to 1.

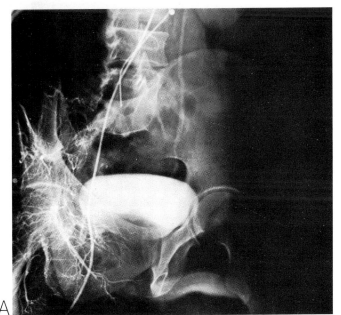
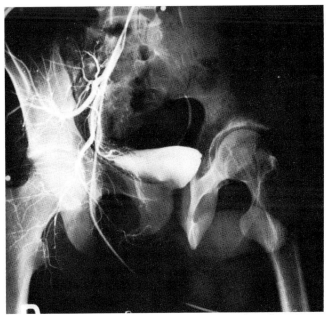

A                                                                                                    B

**Fig. 9.9 A, B.** Superselective arteriography of the arteria pudenda. In A) the pattern is normal, in B) an obstruction of the terminal branches may be noted.

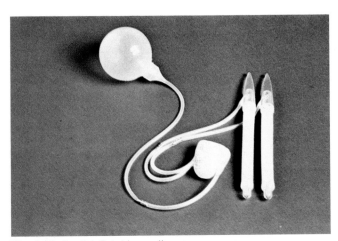

**Fig. 9.10.** Scott inflatable appliance.

For the purposes of identifying vascular impotence, either non-invasive methods are used such as estimation of penile blood pressure (Fig. 9.7) and Doppler flow measurement (Fig. 9.8) or invasive methods such as superselective arteriography of the arteria pudenda (Fig. 9.9 A, B) and cavernography.

Finally, measurement of the bulbocavernous reflex enables us to evaluate the degree of nerve impairment.

The treatment of organic impotence is surgical and consists in the implantation of semirigid or inflatable prostheses.

The latter are undoubtedly more serviceable from the aesthetic and functional points of view, but are based on a hydraulic system (Fig. 9.10) which requires surgical overhaul in one third of cases.

# 10. Stomal problems in handicapped patients

A lucid mind, nimble hands and good eyesight are indispensable requisites for the proper execution of stoma management manoeuvres, but not all ostomy patients are fortunate enough to be so gifted.

In this chapter, in fact, we shall outline the main problems facing patients who lack these attributes.

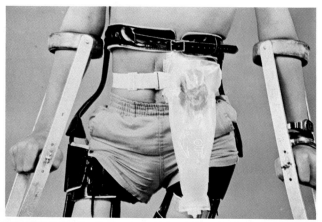

**Fig. 10.1.** Patient suffering from spina bifida. The uretero-colocutaneostomy is prolapsed and sited close to the costal margin. The orthopaedic appliance has been constructed in such a way as not to interfere with the stoma.

## Skeletal deformities and spinal cord lesions

The most important problem here is that deriving from poor siting of the stoma.

When choosing the stoma site, one should bear in mind that these patients are obliged to use orthopaedic appliances (Fig. 10.1) and that their immobility causes them to put on weight (Fig. 10.2 A, B).

The stoma must therefore be clearly visible and easily accessible (Fig. 10.3 A, B), and if the patient is forced to spend a lot of time in a wheel-chair, he must be able to do so without the stoma appliance causing him problems (Fig. 10.4).

Another notable problem in patients with complete medullary section consists in the effects of the loss of sensitivity below the level of the lesion.

The maximum possible care is necessary during stoma management manoeuvres, as any stomal or cutaneous traumas which occur are not perceived by the patient and their effects may become evident only in more advanced stages (Fig. 10.5 A, B, C).

The patient likewise fails to perceive the leakage of urine or faeces and, therefore, to avoid severe, extensive dermatitis, such patients need to be placed under assiduous surveillance.

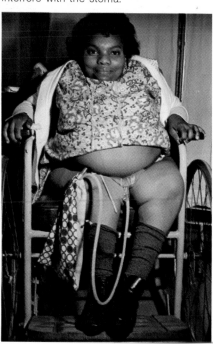
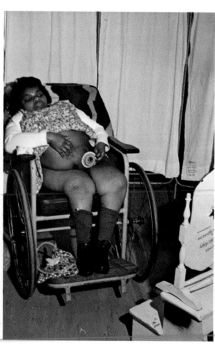

**Fig. 10.2 A, B.** A) Severe congenital kyphoscoliosis. The patient has a colonic urinary conduit. The prolonged state of immobility has produced a substantial increase in weight and the stoma has sunk into the folds of fat. B) To fit the stoma appliance the patient needs to use a mirror.

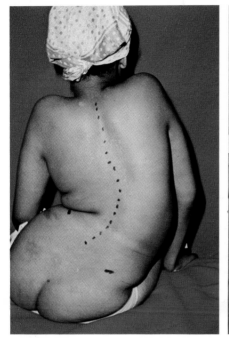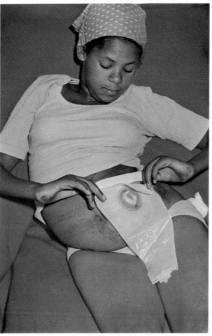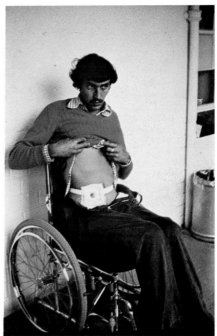

**Fig. 10.3 A, B.** A) Acquired scoliosis in a tetraplegic patient for a fracture of the seventh cervical vertebra. B) The stoma is well sited, clearly visible and easily accessible.

**Fig. 10.4.** Paraplegic patient with urinary diversion for lithiasis of the bladder and recurrent infections. Careful assessment of the habits of the patient, who spends many hours in an invalid chair, made it possible to choose an appropriate stoma site.

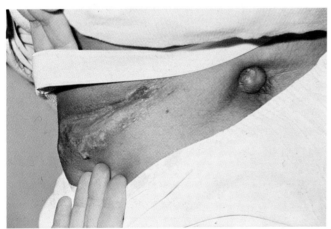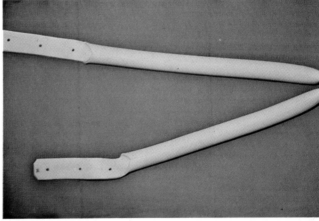

**Fig. 10.5 A, B.** A) Serious traumatic lesion caused by excessively tight urostomy belt in a patient suffering from high medullary section. B) In such cases special tubular belts are recommended.

## Mutilation and functional disablement of the hands

There are many situations which reduce the function of the hand, and in such cases it absolutely essential for the ostomy patient to be able to avail himself of alternative stoma management techniques.

The most common of these techniques is to use mainly the healthy hand and help oneself as best one can with the debilitated hand (Fig. 10.6), but there are cases in which the injured or disabled hand is unusable (Fig. 10.7).

Another method consists in the use of the mouth and teeth (Fig. 10.8 A, B) and there are ostomy patients who develop a surprising degree of ability in this sense and even manage to use relatively complex stoma management systems (Fig. 10.9 A, B, C).

In such patients the use of closed adherent bags is advisable, as drainable bags require more laborious manoeuvres. In cases where the patient cannot do without a drainable bag, the bag used should be of the type equipped with a built-in closing mechanism, as these are more manageable than bags with a movable clip (Fig. 10.10).

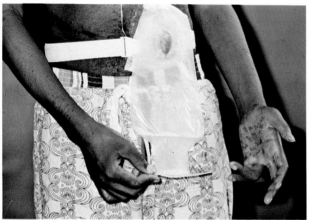

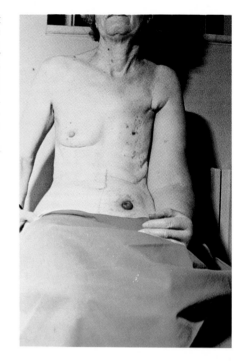

**Fig. 10.7.** Patient with swollen arm after mastectomy. This colostomy patient learnt to do everything with one hand only and showed no hesitation about mastering the irrigation technique.

**Fig. 10.6.** Traumatic lesion of the ulnar nerve with consequent dystrophy and partial functional impotence of the left hand. The patient uses it all the same, albeit with difficulty.

**Fig. 10.8 A, B.** A) Colostomy patient with right hemiplegia. B) The patient uses her mouth to prepare the colostomy appliance.

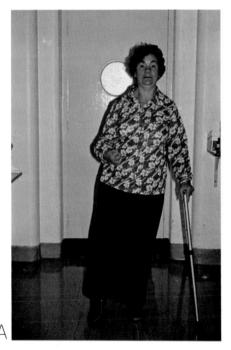

A

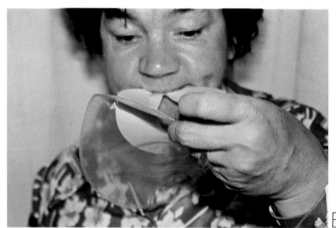

B

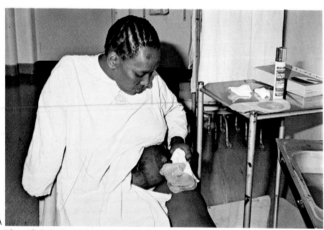

A

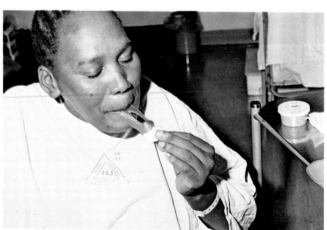

B

**Fig. 10.9 A, B.** A) Amputation of the right forearm owing to a railway accident. The patient performs the clearsing manoeuvres perfectly with her left hand. B) She is able to use karaya rings, which she prepares with her mouth.

PRINTED IN ITALY
BY "BERTONCELLO ARTIGRAFICHE", CITTADELLA (PADOVA)
JANUARY 1983